ICH GUIDELINES ON THALASSEMIA: 2025

ISHBT
Indian Society of Hematology & Blood Transfusion

ICH GUIDELINES ON THALASSEMIA: 2025

INDIAN COLLEGE OF HEMATOLOGY (ICH)

The Academic Wing of ISHBT

Editor

Rabindra Kumar Jena
MD PhD FRCP(London) FICH VTP(USA)
Professor and BMT Physician
Clinical Hematology
SCB Medical College and Hospital
Cuttack, Odisha, India

Associate Editor

Amiya Ranjan Nayak
MBBS(Hons) MD(Gold Medalist) DM
Consultant
Department of Clinical Hemato-Oncology and BMT
Bagchi Sri Shankara Cancer Center and Research Institute
Bhubaneswar, Odisha, India

Nodal Officer

Maitreyee Bhattacharyya
DM(Clinical Hematology, AIIMS)
Director
Department of Hematology
Institute of Hematology and Transfusion Medicine (IHTM)
Kolkata, West Bengal, India

JAYPEE

JAYPEE BROTHERS MEDICAL PUBLISHERS

The Health Sciences Publisher

New Delhi | London

JAYPEE **Jaypee Brothers Medical Publishers (P) Ltd**

Headquarters
EMCA House, 23/23-B
Ansari Road, Daryaganj
New Delhi 110 002, India
Landline: +91-11-23272143, +91-11-23272703
+91-11-23282021, +91-11-23245672
e-mail: jaypee@jaypeebrothers.com

Corporate Office
4838/24, Ansari Road, Daryaganj
New Delhi 110 002, India
Phone: +91-11-43574357
Fax: +91-11-43574314
e-mail: jaypee@jaypeebrothers.com

Overseas Office
JP Medical Ltd.
83, Victoria Street, London
SW1H 0HW (UK)
Phone: +44-20 3170 8910
e-mail: info@jpmedpub.com

EU GPSR Authorised Representative
Logos Europe, 9 rue Nicolas Poussin
17000, La Rochelle, France
Phone: +33 (0) 6 67 93 73 78
e-mail: contact@logoseurope.eu

Website: www.jaypeebrothers.com
Website: www.jaypeedigital.com

Inquiries for bulk sales may be solicited at: jaypee@jaypeebrothers.com

ICH Guidelines on Thalassemia: 2025 / ***Rabindra Kumar Jena***

First Edition: **2026**

ISBN: 978-93-7202-716-7

Printed in India at Sterling Graphics Pvt. Ltd.

Contributors

AK Tripathi MD FRCP(London) FRCP(Glasgow) FRCP(Ireland) FAMS FICP FISHTM FIACM Fellow WHF Fellow NIH(USA) Dean Academics, Professor and Head, Department of Clinical Hematology, King George's Medical University, Lucknow, Uttar Pradesh, India

Amiya Kumar Sahoo MBBS MD DrNB Senior Resident, Department of Clinical Hematology, SCB Medical College and Hospital, Odisha, India

Amiya Ranjan Nayak MBBS(Hons) MD(Gold Medalist) DM Consultant, Department of Clinical Hemato-Oncology and BMT, Bagchi Sri Shankara Cancer Center and Research Institute, Bhubaneswar, Odisha, India

Ashish Dixit MBBS MD DM Senior Consultant Clinical Hematology and Bone Marrow Transplant, Department of Clinical Hematology, Hemato-Oncology and Bone Marrow Transplant, Manipal Hospital, Bengaluru, Karnataka, India

Biplabendu Talukdar MBBS MD PhD(Sc) MPhil(RMTS) MBA(HA) Assistant Professor, Department of IHBT, Medical College Hospital, Kolkata, West Bengal, India

BV Babu PhD Scientist – G and Head, Director In-Charge, Department: Division of Socio-Behavioral, Health Systems and Implementation Research, ICMR, New Delhi, India

Chirasree Sanyal DM(Clinical Hematology) Consultant Hematology and BMT, Department of Hematology, Manipal Hospital, Kolkata, West Bengal, India

Damodar Das MBBS MD Assistant Professor, Department of Clinical Hematology, Gauhati Medical College and Hospital, Guwahati, Assam, India

Jina Bhattacharyya DM(Hematology, AIIMS, Delhi) Professor, Department of Clinical Hematology, Gauhati Medical College and Hospital, Guwahati, Assam, India

JS Arora MSc in Hemoglobinopathy Thalassemiologist, Department of Hematology, University College London, London, United Kingdom

Jyoti Kotwal MD(Pathology) PDF(Hematology) FAMS FRCP(Edinburgh) Chairperson and Professor, Department of Hematology, Sir Ganga Ram Hospital and GRIPMER, New Delhi, India

Jyoti Shaw PhD(Biochemistry, University of Calcutta) ICMR Project Scientist – Level II, Department of Human Genetics Unit, Indian Statistical Institute, Kolkata, West Bengal, India

Maitreyee Bhattacharyya DM(Clinical Hematology, AIIMS) Director, Department of Hematology, Institute of Hematology and Transfusion Medicine (IHTM), Kolkata, West Bengal, India

Manisha Madkaikar MD FNASc Director and Scientist G, Department of Immunohematology, ICMR–National Institute of Immunohematology, Mumbai, Maharashtra, India

Manoranjan Mahapatra MD FRCP FICP FISTM FIACM Professor and Head, Department of Hematology, AIIMS, New Delhi, India

Mukul Aggarwal MBBS MD DM Associate Professor, Department of Hematology, AIIMS, New Delhi, India

Neha Kargutkar PhD(Biochemistry) Postdoctorate Researcher, Department of Clinical and Biological Sciences, University of Turin, Italy

Prashant Sharma MBBS MD DNB DM Professor, Department of Hematology, Postgraduate Institute of Medical Education and Research (PGIMER), Chandigarh, India

Rajendra Chaudhary MD FRCPath Former Professor and Head, Department of Transfusion Medicine, Sanjay Gandhi Postgraduate Institute of Medical Sciences, Lucknow, Uttar Pradesh, India

Rajib De MD DM(Clinical Hematology) Professor, Department of Hematology, NRS Medical College and Hospital, Kolkata, West Bengal, India

Rajib Lochan Sethy DrNB Senior Resident, Department of Clinical Hematology, SCB Medical College and Hospital, Cuttack, Odisha, India

Reena Das MBBS MD DNB Professor and Head, Department of Hematology, Postgraduate Institute of Medical Education and Research (PGIMER), Chandigarh, India

Rabindra Kumar Jena MD PhD FRCP(London) FICH VTP(USA) Professor and BMT Physician, Clinical Hematology, SCB Medical College and Hospital, Cuttack, Odisha, India

Roshan Colah PhD Former Scientist and Director In-Charge, Department of Immunohematology, ICMR–National Institute of Immunohematology, Mumbai, Maharashtra, India

Shailendra Prasad Verma MD(Medicine) DM(Clinical Hematology) Additional Professor and Head, Department of Clinical Hematology, King George's Medical University, Lucknow, Uttar Pradesh, India

Sila Chakrabarti PhD(Biochemistry, Calcutta University) Molecular Biologist, Department of IHTM, Institute of Hematology and Transfusion Medicine (IHTM), Medical College, Kolkata, West Bengal, India

Shipla Roy MBBS MD DM DNB Clinical Tutor, Department of Hematology, NRS Medical College and Hospital, Kolkata, West Bengal, India

Sudha Sethy MBBS MD FICH Associate Professor and Head, Department of Clinical Hematology, SCB Medical College and Hospital, Cuttack, Odisha, India

Sujoy Ghosh DM FRCP Professor, Department of Endocrinology, Institute of Postgraduate Medical Education and Research, Kolkata, West Bengal, India

Sukrita Bhattacharjee MBBS MD DM Consultant, Department of Hematology, Chittaranjan National Cancer Institute, Kolkata, West Bengal, India

Surbhi Dahiya MBBS MD PDF(Hematology) Associate Consultant, Department of Hematology, Sir Ganga Ram Hospital and GRIPMER, New Delhi, India

Sweta Das MBBS MD Fellowship in Clinical Genetics, Consultant Clinical Geneticist, Department of Clinical Genetics, Gauhati Medical College and Hospital Neuberg Center for Genomic Medicine, Guwahati, Assam, India

Tuphan Kanti Dolai DM(Clinical Hematology) AIIMS MD(Medicine) Gold Medalist DNB(Medicine) MBBS FRCP(London) FICP FICH Honorary Secretary of ISHBT, Professor and Head, Department of Hematology, NRS Medical College and Hospital, Kolkata, West Bengal, India

Ved P Choudhry MBBS MD Ex-Head and Professor, Department of Hematology, AIIMS, New Delhi, India

Vikram Mathews MD DM FASc Director, Department of Hematology, Christian Medical College Vellore, Tamil Nadu, India

About Indian College of Hematology

The Indian College of Hematology (ICH) is the academic wing of the Indian Society of Hematology and Blood Transfusion (ISHBT). It represents a conglomeration of hematology leadership in India, with a vision to foster excellence in both clinical and laboratory hematology, enhance quality of health care, and make it accessible across the country.

ICH is committed to:

- Standardizing education and training in hematology
- Establishing evidence-based protocols for diagnosis, management, and control of hematological disorders
- Promoting research, innovation, and collaborative networks across India
- Advising national bodies such as National Medical Commission (NMC) and National Board of Examinations (NBE) on postgraduate education in clinical hematology and hematopathology
- Developing national databases on hematological diseases to guide patient care and policy
- Formulating guidelines, study groups, consensus documents, and recommendations tailored to the Indian context

As part of its academic mission, ICH has taken responsibility for preparing disease-specific guidelines relevant to India. The guidelines on sickle cell disease and anemia have already been released and widely appreciated by healthcare providers, patient groups, and policymakers. Work is in progress on guidelines for thalassemia, hemophilia, aplastic anemia, myeloid leukemias, immune thrombocytopenia (ITP), and stem cell transplantation/CAR T-cell therapy.

These initiatives have been possible due to the cooperation and commitment of ICH fellows and colleagues across the country. With collective efforts, ICH continues to shape the academic and clinical landscape of hematology in India.

We are confident that this Thalassemia Guideline will fulfil its objectives and aspirations.

Long Live ICH!

Rabindra Kumar Jena
Secretary, India College of Hematology
(Academic Wing of ISHBT)

Message from Secretary of Indian College of Hematology

The Indian College of Hematology (ICH) is the academic wing of the Indian Society of Hematology and Blood Transfusion (ISHBT). It is a conglomeration of hematological leadership in India and is driven by the purpose of fostering excellence not only in academic and professional practice involving both clinical hematology and laboratory hematology, but also enhancing the quality of healthcare and making it accessible to people everywhere in the country.

The ICH has a vision to standardize education; establish standard protocols for diagnosis, management, and control of hematological diseases; promote research and development; and address the issues concerning academic excellence and quality of care.

It also aims to act as a national advisory body to give suggestions to National Medical Commission (NMC) and National Board of Examinations (NBE) and allied bodies in all academic and technical activities of postgraduate education in the subjects of clinical hematology and hematopathology, to promote nationwide collaborative research and prepare databases for various hematological diseases, and to formulate the different guidelines, study groups, consensus documents, recommendations and research groups, and other academic activities as assigned by ISHBT. ICH in collaboration with the Indian Council of Medical Research (ICMR) prepared and released national guidelines on the management and control of sickle cell disease which is India specific and will benefit all stakeholders. The National Guideline on Nutritional Anemia in India by ICH has already been released and well appreciated by all stakeholders.

The present guideline on Thalassemia is in the line of our commitment. I am sure this is going to benefit all concerned including policy makers, regulatory bodies, patient groups, nongovernmental organizations (NGOs), healthcare givers, etc.

Rabindra Kumar Jena
Secretary, ICH

Message from Honorary Secretary of Indian Society of Hematology and Blood Transfusion

The Indian Society of Hematology and Blood Transfusion (ISHBT) conducts several works in advancing hematology and blood transfusion through its annual conferences, publications like the Indian Journal of Hematology and Blood Transfusion (IJHBT), collaborations with international bodies, developing guidelines for hematological disorders, and academic programs. It also provides support to researchers and clinicians, offers awards to encourage excellence, contributes to social outreach programs, and published a consensus document for managing hematological diseases.

The Indian College of Hematology (ICH) is an academic wing of ISHBT working in formulating various guidelines of hematological disorders to facilitate better practice of hematology across nation. Through advocacy meetings with government stakeholders, ISHBT is helping to provide a forum for discussing the present hematology-concerning issues and coming forth with better healthcare practices. Recently, ICH in collaboration with the Indian Council of Medical Research (ICMR) and other societies has prepared and published guidelines on sickle cell and also published guidelines in nutritional anemia.

Thalassemia is the most common hematological disorder and a burning public health issue across India. ISHBT has devised this in India in the Guidelines for Diagnosis and Management of Thalassemia. This guideline is going to aid the medical practitioners and stakeholders, and most importantly it will help in better patient care management.

With this guideline, India will become a nation free from thalassemia one day.

Tuphan Kanti Dolai
DM(Clinical Hematology) AIIMS
MD(Medicine) Gold Medalist DNB(Medicine) MBBS FRCP(London) FICP FICH
Honorary Secretary of ISHBT
Professor and Head, Department of Hematology
NRS Medical College and Hospital
Kolkata, West Bengal, India

Preface

We have entered an era where thalassemia, once considered as a fatal disease, is now preventable, manageable, and even curable. This has become possible because of better understanding of disease biology, transfusion services, newer disease-modifying drugs, and progress of stem cell transplant. This has increased the survival of patients, decreased their morbidity, and improved the quality of life of thalassemia patients significantly.

However, the situation may not be that bright in developing countries like India because of lack of awareness about the disease, problem of access to healthcare facilities, cultural and social background of the patients, and financial constraints.

The Indian College of Hematology (ICH) commits to supporting patient and parent organizations, healthcare professionals, and policymakers. These guidelines are a cornerstone of our mission to help the nation to control and treat thalassemia. This guideline will serve as resources for healthcare providers and a document which helps the policymakers to formulate a national guideline.

The document envisages the avenues possible to expand the reach of the program in terms of:

- Awareness generation on thalassemia
- Screening of the target population for thalassemia
- Provision of prenatal diagnostic services for thalassemia
- Comprehensive care for thalassemia
- Promoting education, research, awareness, and advocacy

This guideline offers quality and evidence-based information for clinicians and other health professionals to help them in their effort to provide the best possible treatment to the patients under their care. Thalassemia often leads to iron overload and multiple organ involvement requiring involvement and expert opinion of health professionals at several levels and different specialties. It is because of this reason that this guideline included health professionals of various disciplines and emphasized the need for multidisciplinary care.

I am grateful for the sincere efforts of ICH to improve the situation. We humbly request governments to provide support to the unmet needs of patients with this disorder. We encourage healthcare professionals to follow this guideline for prevention, diagnosis, and management of patients at their centers. Evidence-based practices outlined in these guidelines are vital for enabling early diagnosis, effective management, and timely intervention. They also serve as a roadmap for integrating novel therapies and thus ensuring that all thalassemia patients, irrespective of location, culture, religion, and language, have access to optimal standards of care—a basic and fundamental human right.

Another aim of this guideline is to promote research activities with translational values. Research also increases the number of stakeholders that the thalassemia patient requires for a better life. Apart from the clinicians, basic science, pharmaceutical industries, and nongovernmental organizations contribute a lot for the proper care of thalassemia patients and should be a part of any guideline and national policies.

The development of a group of expert medical specialists allows sharing of knowledge through networking at the national level. The establishment of centers of excellence and special dedicated thalassemia care centers for these patients has been shown to improve care, and such centers can become reference centers to refer cases for periodic monitoring and troubleshooting. This concept of sharing expertise is particularly important in India.

This guideline was made by experts with decades of experience in thalassemia prevention, diagnosis, and management. I extend my heartfelt gratitude to all the authors whose dedication and expertise have made it possible to formulate the guideline.

Maitreyee Bhattacharyya
Rabindra Kumar Jena

Contents

1

CHAPTER

Epidemiology and Burden of Thalassemia

Amiya Ranjan Nayak, Rajib Lochan Sethy, Rabindra Kumar Jena

INTRODUCTION

Thalassemia is a common inherited hemoglobin disorder caused by mutations in the α, β, or δ globin genes, leading to reduced hemoglobin synthesis and ineffective erythropoiesis. It includes α-, β-, δβ-, and rarer forms like γδβ-thalassemia, with α- and β-thalassemia being most prevalent. Clinical severity ranges from asymptomatic carriers to transfusion-dependent β-thalassemia (TDT), the most severe form, requiring lifelong transfusions and iron chelation to prevent complications like organ damage and endocrine dysfunction.[1] Untreated severe β-thalassemia can be fatal early in life. The WHO identifies thalassemia as a major global health issue, with over 40,000 births annually affected by β-thalassemia, about 25,500 of which are TDT.[2] Outcomes vary widely between high- and low-income countries, with higher childhood mortality in resource-limited settings. Though government initiatives now provide free blood transfusions and iron chelation therapy in several states, comprehensive care remains unaffordable for many families due to additional medical costs. While bone marrow transplantation offers a potential cure, its high cost and limited accessibility restrict its use.

Global Burden

Thalassemia remains a major global health challenge, affecting over 13 million individuals worldwide in 2021, with nearly 120,000 new cases reported annually. It spans all age groups and is present in 204 countries, though prevalence varies by region.[3] Over the past few decades, incidence and prevalence rates have gradually declined, largely due to the implementation of prenatal screening, genetic counseling, and assisted reproductive technologies such as in vitro fertilization with preimplantation genetic diagnosis. These efforts have significantly reduced the number of births with thalassemia.

Despite a global reduction in mortality and disability-adjusted life years (DALYs) associated with thalassemia, the disease continues to impose a considerable burden, especially among children. Hemoglobinopathies, including thalassemia, are responsible for 3.4% of global deaths in children under five, and 6.4% in Africa alone.[2] Although traditionally concentrated in the Mediterranean, Middle East, and Southeast Asia, thalassemia is now increasingly seen in non-endemic areas like Western Europe and North America due to migration.[4] This shift presents new healthcare demands and financial strains. Managing TDT over a patient's lifetime can cost between $5 and 5.7 million, primarily driven by iron chelation and transfusion costs.[5] Optimizing chelation therapy could cut these expenses by up to one-third. As life expectancy improves, especially in patients aged 50–69, there is a growing incidence of long-term complications, notably cardiac issues, underscoring the importance of ongoing surveillance, patient awareness, and access to cost-effective, comprehensive care.

EPIDEMIOLOGY OF THALASSEMIA IN INDIA

In India, thalassemia is a serious public health issue that impacts millions of people from the country's diverse population. According to estimates, 3–4% of people, or 35–45 million people, are carriers of beta thalassemia; rates can reach 17% in some ethnic groups (Sindhis, Lohanas, Bhanushalis, Prajapatis, Banias, Jains, Patels in western India).[6] Significant diversity in carrier frequency has been found by regional research, even within small regions of Gujarat and Maharashtra. Hemoglobin variations like HbE and HbS are also highly prevalent in some areas and communities, especially among underprivileged and tribal populations. It is usual for these variations to be co-inherited. As per ICMR data published in 2022, there are an estimated 42 million carriers and > 12000 newborns born each year with a substantial and clinically severe hemoglobinopathy. The total number of affected individuals in the country is estimated to be between 100,000 and 150,000.[7]

Alpha-thalassemia carrier rates in India show considerable variation. Among non-tribal populations, the average prevalence is about 13%, ranging between 3 and 23% in different communities. In tribal groups, the prevalence is significantly higher, ranging from 17 up to 97%.[8]

Hemoglobin E (HbE) is especially widespread in the northeastern states like Assam, Meghalaya, and Tripura, where carrier frequencies range from 20 to 64%. In eastern India, particularly in West Bengal, the prevalence of HbE carriers is between 3 and 10%. The combination of HbE and beta-thalassemia is the most frequently observed hemoglobin disorder in these regions. Moreover, over 50 rare alpha- and beta-globin chain variants have been documented in India, with the possibility of more yet to be identified.[9]

MUTATIONAL LANDSCAPE OF THALASSEMIA IN INDIA

With more than 80 distinct mutations found in different parts of India, the range of beta-thalassemia variants is extremely varied. Despite this variation, >95% of all severe cases of beta-thalassemia in the Indian population are caused by five mutations that are very prevalent. These include: IVS-I-5 (G>C), IVS-I-1 (G>T), 619 bp deletion, Codons 8/9 (+G), Codons 41/42 (–TTCT).[10]

In the case of alpha-thalassemia, the most frequently observed genetic defect is the $-\alpha3.7$ gene deletion, followed by the $-\alpha4.2$ deletion. Other deletions such as the polyadenylation signal mutation, --SA (South African), --SEA (Southeast Asian), and --MED (Mediterranean) types have also been reported but are relatively rare.[8]

Diagnosing some beta-thalassemia carriers can be difficult due to borderline HbA2 levels and near-normal red cell indices. In northern India, the Cap +1 (A>C) mutation is relatively common and often presents with such borderline values. Additionally, certain common beta-thal mutations like IVS-I-5 (G>C), codon 15 (G>A), and codon 30 (G>C) may also show normal HbA2 levels.[11] Coinheritance of delta-globin gene mutations with beta-thal mutations can further lower HbA2 levels, leading to diagnostic challenges and possible misclassification of carriers as normal.

ECONOMIC BURDEN

In India, thalassemia places a heavy financial strain on families and the healthcare system. TDT is mostly treated with iron chelation therapy and frequent blood transfusions. The average yearly treatment cost, according to a study conducted at a tertiary care facility in North India, is approximately INR 74,948 (US$1,135), with a significant variation based on the patient's age. Managing a single thalassemia patient typically costs a family up to 39% of their income.[12] Annual blood needs are expected to increase from 4.5 to 8.25 million units between 2016 and 2026, and treatment expenses may jump from INR 30 to 55 billion.[13] Numerous studies understate the true expenses, particularly in cases where therapy is not at its best and access to high-quality transfusion services is still restricted in rural areas. Additionally, the emotional and social costs—such as the shame and worse quality of life that patients and their families endure—are rarely included in economic evaluations.

Even though more than 35 hospitals are able to provide hematopoietic stem cell transplantation (HSCT), the treatment is still not widely used in India, where just 250 procedures are carried out each year. With a matched sibling donor, a successful HSCT can cost anywhere between INR 10 and 15 lakh (US$15,500–23,000).[14,15] With a higher quality of life and reduced long-term expenses, HSCT is more economical than a lifetime of transfusions and chelation, despite its high initial cost. Numerous government programs and corporate social responsibility initiatives offer financial assistance, which may help increase access to this treatment alternative.

STATE WISE PREVALENCE OF BETA THALASSEMIA TRAIT (ICMR DATA 2022)

The ICMR 2022 data on state-wise prevalence of the beta-thalassemia trait provides a broad overview of regional variability across India **(Table 1)**. However, these figures must be interpreted with caution, as they do not accurately represent the national scenario. The data is derived from a heterogeneous mix of studies—some are population-based, others stem from newborn screening programs, hospital records, or are limited to specific tribal or non-tribal communities. In the absence of a uniform, nationwide population screening program, these prevalence estimates, while useful for highlighting high-risk regions, fall short of capturing the true burden of beta-thalassemia in the country.

CONCLUSION AND FUTURE PERSPECTIVE

Given India's immense genetic diversity and the widespread prevalence of hemoglobinopathies, there is an urgent need for well-structured thalassemia prevention programs. With an estimated 42 million carriers and over 12,000 children born annually with severe hemoglobinopathies such as TDT, the burden on families and the healthcare system is both profound and escalating. Regional data from the ICMR (2022) reveal striking variability in carrier frequencies, particularly among certain ethnic and tribal populations, yet these figures only hint at the broader reality due to the absence of a uniform national screening initiative. Current management strategies, though bolstered by government schemes offering free transfusion and chelation, remain economically unsustainable for many, especially in rural and underserved regions. In contrast, global experiences highlight how prenatal screening, genetic counseling, and public awareness campaigns have successfully reduced disease incidence. Thus, India must prioritize a comprehensive prevention framework that includes carrier detection, public education, premarital and antenatal screening, and genetic counseling, integrated into both rural and urban healthcare systems. Such programs

TABLE 1: State wise prevalence of beta thalassemia trait as per ICMR 2022 data (Atlas of Hemoglobinopathies in India).

State	Prevalence	State	Prevalence
Western region		**North Eastern region**	
Maharashtra	0.10–21.20%	Assam	0.42–8.64%
Gujarat	0.7–15.59%	Arunachal Pradesh	HbE trait 5.61–35.13%
Rajasthan	2.5–7.60%	Meghalaya	HbE trait 4.5–41.30%
Goa	2 reports	Manipur	HbE trait 0.99–4.33%
Dadra and Nagar haveli	1.09–2.36%	Tripura	0.11–39.49%
Southern region		**Northern region**	
Andhra Pradesh	5.3% (one study)	Delhi	2.9–56.36%
Telangana	21% (one study)	Punjab	3.3–4.1%
Karnataka	5.2–33%	Haryana	3.5–7.4%
Tamil Nadu	0.11–37%	Uttar Pradesh	2.8–58.6%
Kerala	NA	Uttarakhand	1.5–3.21%
Eastern region		Himachal Pradesh	2.1–5.80%
West Bengal	2.59–8.3%	Jammu and Kashmir	3.05–13.90%
Odisha	0.50–8.50%	**Central region**	
Jharkhand	10–14.94%	Chhattisgarh	NA
Bihar	4.81% (one study)	Madhya Pradesh	1.8–20.50%
Andaman and Nicobar Islands	3.44–7.80%		

not only promise to curb the birth of affected children but also reduce the long-term clinical and financial burden of thalassemia on individuals and the nation.

SUMMARY

- Thalassemia is a genetic blood disorder primarily caused by mutations in α-, β-, or δ-globin genes, leading to reduced hemoglobin production and ineffective erythropoiesis.
- The disease spectrum ranges from asymptomatic carriers to severe transfusion-dependent β-thalassemia (TDT), which requires lifelong blood transfusions and iron chelation to avoid complications like organ damage.
- Globally, over 13 million people are affected, with around 120,000 new cases annually, including over 40,000 new births with β-thalassemia, making it a major public health challenge.
- Mortality and disability due to thalassemia have decreased in many regions due to improved prenatal screening and genetic counseling, yet the burden remains high, especially in low-resource countries.
- India has a high carrier burden, with 3–4% of its population (~ 42 million) carrying β-thalassemia traits, and over 12,000 babies born annually with severe forms.
- Certain Indian communities and regions (e.g., Sindhis, northeastern states, tribal populations) show carrier rates as high

as 64% for some hemoglobinopathies like HbE.

- Five common mutations account for over 95% of severe β-thalassemia cases in India, while over 80 mutations have been reported nationwide, contributing to diagnostic complexity.
- The economic burden is substantial, with annual treatment costs averaging INR 75,000 per patient, consuming up to 39% of a family's income, and national transfusion needs rising steadily.
- Curative treatment via hematopoietic stem cell transplantation (HSCT) exists but is limited by cost, donor availability, and access, with only about 250 procedures done annually in India.
- India urgently needs a comprehensive thalassemia prevention strategy, including national carrier screening, premarital and prenatal counseling, and public awareness to reduce the future disease burden.

REFERENCES

1. Kattamis A, Kwiatkowski JL, Aydinok Y. Thalassaemia. Lancet. 2022;399(10343):2310-24.
2. Modell B, Darlison M. Global epidemiology of haemoglobin disorders and derived service indicators. Bull World Health Organ. 2008;86(6):480-7.
3. Tuo Y, Li Y, Li Y, et al. Global, regional, and national burden of thalassemia, 1990-2021: a systematic analysis for the global burden of disease study 2021. EClinicalMedicine. 2024;72:102619.
4. De Sanctis V, Kattamis C, Canatan D, et al. β-thalassemia distribution in the old world: an ancient disease seen from a historical standpoint. Mediterr J Hematol Infect Dis. 2017;9(1).
5. Udeze C, Maruszczyk K, Atter M, et al. PB2339: projected lifetime economic burden of transfusion dependent beta-thalassemia in the United States. Hemasphere. 2022;6(Suppl):2208-9.
6. Madan N, Sharma S, Sood SK, et al. Frequency of b thalassemia trait and other hemoglobinopathies in northern and western India. Indian J Hum Genet. 2010;16:16-25.
7. Kantharaj A, Chandrashekar S. Coping with the burden of thalassemia: aiming for a thalassemia free world. Glob J Transfus Med. 2018;3(1):1-5.
8. Nadkarni A, Phanasgaonkar S, Colah R, et al. Prevalence and molecular characterization of alpha-thalassemia syndromes among Indians. Genet Test. 2008;12(2):177-80.
9. Colah RB, Seth T. Thalassemia in India. Hemoglobin. 2022;46(1):20-6.
10. Panigrahi I, Marwaha RK. Mutational spectrum of thalassemias in India. Indian J Hum Genet. 2007;13(1):36-7.
11. Gorivale M, Sawant P, Mehta P, et al. Challenges in prenatal diagnosis of beta thalassaemia: couples with normal HbA2 in one partner. Prenat Diagn. 2015;35(13):1353-7.
12. Moirangthem A, Phadke SR. Socio-demographic profile and economic burden of treatment of transfusion dependent thalassemia. Indian J Pediatr. 2018;85(2):102-7.
13. Sinha S, Seth T, Colah RB, et al. Haemoglobinopathies in India: estimates of blood requirements and treatment costs for the decade 2017-2026. J Community Genet. 2020;11(1): 39-45.
14. Mathews V, Balasubramanian P, Abraham A, et al. Allogeneic stem cell transplant for thalassemia major in India. Pediatr Hematol Oncol J. 2017;2(4):114-20.
15. Kulkarni U, George B. Access to hematopoietic stem-cell trans plantation in India. J Postgrad Med. 2019;65(1):1-4.

2

CHAPTER

Laboratory Diagnosis of Thalassemia

Jyoti Kotwal, Surbhi Dahiya

INTRODUCTION

Thalassemia, a hereditary hemoglobinopathy characterized by defective synthesis of globin chains, poses a significant public health challenge in India. With an estimated 10,000 children born annually with thalassemia major and a carrier prevalence ranging from 3 to 17% across various regions, the burden of this disorder necessitates a robust and standardized approach to screening, diagnosis, and prevention. Recognizing the critical need for early detection and genetic counseling, the Government of India and various health authorities have initiated comprehensive guidelines for thalassemia testing. These protocols aim to streamline diagnostic practices, ensure quality control in laboratory procedures, and promote equitable access to screening services—particularly among high-risk populations and in antenatal care settings.

This chapter outlines the recommended screening methodologies, diagnostic algorithms, laboratory standards, and ethical considerations. It serves as a reference for clinicians, laboratory personnel, public health professionals, and policymakers engaged in the prevention and management of hemoglobinopathies.

Two distinct methods of screening and diagnosis are used in laboratory investigations of thalassemia. Screening aims at the use of algorithms and risk assessments considering ethnicity etc., to pick up maximum cases of thalassemia/hemoglobinopathies in a cost-effective manner while reducing the number of false positive and false negative findings. The presumptive diagnosis must be based on at least two different but complimentary techniques. Definitive diagnosis requires more thorough investigation and is now increasingly using molecular techniques to improve accuracy.[1]

LAB DIAGNOSIS COMES INTO PLAY

- To confirm a provisional clinical diagnosis of transfusion dependent thalassemia (TDT) which was earlier classified as beta thalassemia major and intermedia
- To provide an explanation for a hematological anomaly like microcytosis or anemia
- Preconception and antenatal screening of parents
- To permit genetic counseling of prospective parents
- Clinics carrying out assisted conceptions must always perform relevant screening and testing as per the necessity.

Antenatal Screening and Testing

- Antenatal screening should be performed for thalassemia, sickle cell diseases and other clinically relevant hemoglobinopathies like, compound heterozygous states or homozygous states with thalassemia and sickle cell diseases.

- Thalassemia diagnoses require a combination of laboratory tests including the measurement of red blood cell indices by automatic hematology analyzer, Hb subtype analysis, and quantification of HbA2 and HbF.
- A minimum of two methods, each based on distinct but complimentary ideas, must serve as the basis for presumptive identification.
- The high-performance liquid chromatography (HPLC) or capillary zone electrophoresis (CE) system can distinguish thalassemic diseases and the carriers in a rapid manner. These systems give both qualitative and quantitative analyses of Hb components with good precision and reproducibility. They have enabled us to do both prenatal and postnatal diagnoses of thalassemia within a few minutes.
- Since they are recessive conditions, hematological testing is necessary and makes carrier identification possible.
- Iron-deficiency anemia must be ruled out because carriers of either α- or β-thalassemia (heterozygotes) exhibit microcytic hypochromic parameters with or without anemia.
- The family history and ethnicity may offer valuable insights into the laboratory diagnosis of thalassemias following ferritin measurement.
- The foundation for identifying a thalassemia carrier is the hematological parameters, such as red cell indices and morphology, followed by the separation and analysis of Hb fractions **(Table 1)**.
- The most used formulas based on red cell indices are the following:
  Mentzer index (MI) = MCV/RBC
  Discriminant factor (DF) = MCV × (RDW/Hb × 100)
  Shine and Lal index (S and L) = MCV × (MCH/100)

TABLE 1: Utilizing combination of automated CBC based red cell indices and Hb HPLC report as an aid to screening for thalassemia trait.

Mean corpuscular volume in fL	Mean corpuscular Hb in pg	RBC count	Red cell distribution width CV(%)	Hb-HPLC	Possible diagnosis
>80	>27	Normal	12–18	HbA2 < 3.5% HbF normal	Normal
<80	< 27	Raised/high normal	12–18	HbA2 > 3.5% HbF < 2%	β-thalassemia trait
<80	<27	Raised/high normal	12–18	HbA2 <3.5% HbF < 2%	Silent β-thalassemia
<80	<27	Raised/high normal	12–18	HbA2 < 2% +/– HbH	α-thalassemia trait
<80	<27	Raised/high normal	12–18	HbA decreased HbA2 decreased HbF increased	δβ-thalassemia trait
<80	<27	Normal/low	>18	HbA2<3.5% HbF<2%	Iron deficiency anemia
<80	<27	Raised/ high normal	12–18	Hb S, D, E, etc.	Other hemoglobinopathy

Srivastava index (SI) = MCH/RBC
RDW index (RDWI) = (MCV × RDW)/RBC^2

- Studies have shown that low MCV with normal RDW CV% and high TRBC (total red cell counts) on cell counters to favor thalassemia trait over iron deficiency, however, as many Indian women have concomitant iron deficiency, the western cut-off of RDW CV approximately 16% does not work. Because considerable overlap has been seen, it is advised to utilize at least two cutoff points when using these calculations to differentiate between iron deficiency and thalassemia. In an Indian study on 640 adults with microcytosis (MCV <80 fL), the cut-off values obtained were MCV ≤76 fL, total red blood cell count ≥4.9 × 10^{12}/L and red cell distribution width ≤18%. These were different from those observed in the West, possibly because of the high prevalence of iron deficiency in India.[3]
- The use of MCV <80 fL and MCH < 27 pg is a useful method to start with the screening based on CBC reports and advise further testing with HPLC/CE in all antenatal cases.[4]
- If the MCH is < 27 pg consider HbA2 percentage for the diagnosis of β thalassemia heterozygosity and HbF percentage for the diagnosis of δβ thalassemia heterozygosity.
- If MCH < 27 pg consider the following possibilities:
    - HbA2 (%) >3.5%: β thalassemia trait
    - HbF (%) ≥5%: Consider the δβ thalassemia trait.
    - HbA2 (%) <3.5%: Look for co-existing δ thalassemia as it may reduce HbA2 into normal range. Also perform iron studies as it may be a case of iron deficiency with thalassemia trait. Repeat after correction of iron deficiency.
    - HbA2 (%) ≥8%: Consider Hb Lepore; ≥15%: Consider HbE trait
- If MCH is normal with HbA2 ≥4%: Consider the milder form of β thalassemia trait.
- If MCH is normal with ≥10% of HbF: Consider HPFH.
- HbA2 between 3 and 3.5% is borderline and with low MCV and MCH can be seen in alpha, delta, beta thalassemia, normal HbA2 β thalassemia. These need molecular testing for confirmation of diagnosis.
- Care must be taken for variants co-eluting with HbA2 like Hb Lepore, Hb D-Iran and HbE. Heterozygous Hb D-Iran have significantly higher Hb, MCV, MCH, and MCHC on hemogram and the mean peak area of the HbA2 window is usually ≥40% with retention time range of 3.57 ± 0.048. While HbE has retention time range of 3.70 ± 0.026 with peak area of ≤30%. Hb Lepore has RT of 3.37 s with peak area of approximately 12.1 ± 1.5% and has a characteristic hump on its downward peak.
- If MCH is less than 27 pg, alpha thalassemia carrier status should be taken into consideration after ruling out the other options.
- Although homozygous α^+ thalassemia is not a clinically significant disorder but causes diagnostic dilemmas with iron deficiency states. However, for antenatal screening, further assessment is warranted irrespective of the iron status due to insufficient time to reassess the indices after iron therapy.
- When MCH is less than 25 pg, the likelihood of α^0 thalassemia, which is uncommon in India, should be evaluated based on family history. This must be verified by the mother's DNA and, if necessary, the father's as well.
- Compound heterozygosity of triplicate alpha-globin gene deletion with beta-thalassemia trait can lead to a range of clinical manifestations, from mild anemia to thalassemia intermedia symptoms and requires early diagnosis with DNA analysis.

- HbA with an abnormal band must be evaluated for HbS, HbC, HbD and all others as per retention time HPLC or zone on CE.
- A supplemental method suitable for the suspected anomaly should be used to confirm abnormal laboratory screening results.
- While using red cell indices in pregnant women we need to remember that the MCV increases by 3 fL and total RBC count decreases as part of normal physiology of pregnancy and the indices like Mentzer's are not good for screening.
- HbA2 > 3.5% and HbF above 5% in pregnancy needs further investigation -whichever of these systems is used (EU FDA approved method should be used)
- Delaying the investigation for hemoglobinopathies in pregnant women while treating iron deficiency presumptively is not justified because it will take longer to find at-risk carrier couples who could receive a prenatal diagnosis.
- Thus, every antenatal woman not tested earlier should undergo Hb-HPLC. If possible, the testing should be finished before 10 weeks of pregnancy, and the entire procedure, including any necessary testing of the baby's biological father, should be finished within the first 16 weeks.[5]
- Testing should be performed on women who present for the first time late in pregnancy since the results will be useful for this and subsequent pregnancies and will allow the healthcare provider to provide genetic counseling regarding future pregnancies.
- *Partner screening* in a high prevalence population for antenatal women partners, samples may be collected for early decision on prenatal diagnosis of homozygous or double heterozygous thalassemia after proper genetic counseling.
- However, there are certain conditions not detected by the antenatal screening program:
    - Silent/near silent β thalassemia carriers (**Table 2**—atypical β thalassemia carriers—genotype and phenotype)
    - α^0 thalassemia carriers in non-prevalent areas.
    - Dominant hemoglobinopathy in the biological father with the mother of the baby having normal screen.

TABLE 2: The atypical phenotype of β thalassemia trait with reduced MCV and MCH and raised HbA2 may be modified by several genetic and acquired factors causing problems in carrier identification.[6]

Phenotype	Genotype
Normal MCV and MCH and high HbA2	Coinheritance of α thalassemia
Reduced MCV and MCH, borderline HbA2	• Some mild β thalassemia alleles • Coinheritance of α thalassemia • δβ thalassemia
Normal MCV, MCH with borderline/normal HbA2	• Very mild/silent alleles • Triplicated α globulin gene • KLF1 mutations
Very low MCV, MCH with low Hb and severe phenotype	• Coinheritance of α-gene defects • HbH disease and triple α locus • Genotype α-/-α • Hyper unstable globulins

  - Co-inheritance of β thalassemia and triplicated α in a newborn.
  - Some uncommon but clinically significant hemoglobinopathies.
  - Thalassemia carriers masked by vitamin B12/folate deficiency, liver disease, iron deficiency etc. (**Table 3**—causes of raised and reduced HbA2 levels).

When to do Prenatal Testing

- The National Health Mission Guidelines for hemoglobinopathies in India, clearly lays down the requisites for pre-natal diagnosis and must be carried out in "at risk" couples after proper genetic counseling and written informed consent. The chorionic villous sampling should be performed within 10–12 weeks, amniocentesis only after 18 weeks and fetal blood testing (cordocentesis) within 18–20 weeks.[5]

When to do Newborn Screening

- All newborns should be screened for sickle cell diseases, *β thalassemia major, transfusion dependent thalassemia, hemoglobin H disease and HbE with β thalassemia. When required, diagnosis should be made on their parents' HPLC and red cell indices in an appropriate family history, ethnic background and DNA analysis as per the requirements.*

What to do for the Evaluation of Microcytosis Outside of Antenatal Screening?

- Additional testing for iron deficiency and anemia of chronic disease should be conducted when microcytosis is evaluated outside of antenatal screening. Repeating HPLC after iron deficiency correction is recommended because severe iron deficiency anemia (Hb<8 g/L) can lower the HbA2 level by as much as 0.5%.
- New cell counters provide parameters like Hypo-He and Micro-R that can be used to calculate the Urrechaga index (% MicroR – % Hypo-He – RDW with cutoff of –7.6.) that has proven to be the most reliable index with sensitivity of 100%, for recognizing thalassemia carriers.[7]

TABLE 3: Causes of raised HbA2 and low HbA2 that help in interpretation of screening tests.

Condition	Increased HbA2 (Potential causes)	Decreased HbA2 (Potential causes)
Inherited	Beta thalassemia β-thalassemia trait (heterozygosity)	α-thalassemia α-thalassemia trait (α^+ and α^0)
	Deletional HPFH (some types, especially Vietnamese/South East Asian)	δβ-thalassemia
	Co-inheritance of β-thalassemia with α-thalassemia	Hemoglobin Lepore
	Sickle cell trait (increased HbA2 on HPLC due to Hb S1d)	Silent β-thalassemia alleles
	Co-inheritance of β- and δ-thalassemia	
Acquired	Megaloblastic anemia (folate/B12 deficiency)	Severe iron deficiency
	Antiretroviral therapy (NRTIs) and HIV	Sideroblastic anemia
	Some other hemoglobinopathies/variants (e.g., Hb S1d in sickle cell)	Anemia of chronic disease
	Hyperthyroidism (Thyrotoxicosis)	Lead poisoning
	Leukemias	Aplastic anemia
		Hypothyroidism

- HbA2 levels exceeding 4% with normal indices may suggest the presence of β thalassemia trait, potentially in conjunction with α thalassemia. Re-analyze the CBC, repeat the HbA2, and look for causes such as vitamin B12/folate insufficiency, medications, liver disease/alcohol, or HIV infection.
- Regardless of the pattern of red cell indices, hemoglobinopathy evaluation should be taken into consideration in any case of unexplained microcytosis.

Transfusion-dependent Thalassemia/ Beta-thalassemia Major and Intermedia

- Between 6 and 24 months of life, β-thalassemia major typically manifests clinically as severe microcytic/normocytic anemia, moderate jaundice, and hepatosplenomegaly. The hematological diagnosis is predicated on extremely low MCH (<20 pg) and a decreased hemoglobin level (<7 g/dL). Severe erythrocyte morphologic alterations are visible in the peripheral blood smear, including target cells, a large number of erythroblasts, poikilocytosis, and basophilic stippling. The degree of ineffective erythropoiesis is correlated with the number of erythroblasts.[1,8]
- When hemoglobin analysis is performed on the traditional form of β-thalassemia major (homozygotes β°), HbF accounts for 92–95% of total hemoglobin with absent HbA. In double heterozygosity(β°/β^+) cases, the HbA levels range between 10 and 30% and HbF between 70 and 90%. Under such circumstances, both parents typically exhibit β-carrier-typical hematological parameters.
- In a post-transfused, transfusion dependent thalassemia (TDT) the HbF may not be high, and parental screening is required for diagnosis; both parents will have thalassemia trait.
- The clinical spectrum of thalassemia intermedia and the hematological phenotype is very wide.
- Patients with milder forms may have moderate-to-mild anemia, and the levels of HbA and HbF are very much dependent on the underlying molecular defects and the degree of ineffective erythropoiesis. These patients are usually capable of surviving without regular blood transfusions. Hb levels are greater than 7 g/dL, even in patients with more severe forms of thalassemia intermedia, and they may decrease in the event of concurrent events like infection, surgery, or pregnancy. When feasible, family studies are very beneficial since they enable the assessment of hematological differences in carriers.[9]
- Since they may have β^+ homozygosity, β^0 heterozygosity, or double heterozygosity with α thalassemia, HbE, or sickle trait, molecular analysis is still the gold standard for diagnosing thalassemia intermedia phenotype.
- Thus, all cases for diagnosis need to be worked up for thalassemia syndromes, e.g., HbE syndromes, HbE- β thalassemia, HbS- β thalassemia HbS- δβ thalassemia, Hbs-HPFH, etc., and family studies and molecular studies help in final diagnosis.[4,10]

Laboratory Methods Utilized in Screening and Diagnosing Hemoglobinopathies

- *High-performance liquid chromatography*:
  - Usually it distinguishes hemoglobin A, A2, F, S, C, D-Punjab and G-Philadelphia from each other. Although Hb E and Hb Lepore co-elute with A2 (as other hemoglobins co-elute with A, S and F), they can be identified by other techniques.
  - HPLC has the drawback of separating unmodified hemoglobin from

glycosylated and other derivative forms of hemoglobin, which can complicate interpretation. For instance, hemoglobin S derivatives may co-elute with hemoglobin A2, making its measurement imprecise.[11]

- *Capillary electrophoresis*:
  - It can be used for the quantification of hemoglobins A, S, A2 and F and for the detection, provisional identification and quantification of many variant hemoglobins.
  - CE is appropriate for diagnosing beta thalassemia trait since it typically yields an accurate measurement of HbA2. It allows for the precise measurement of HbA2 in the presence of HbE (but not HbC) and isolates HbE from HbA2 **(Figs. 1A and B).**[12]
  - It does not separate glycated fractions, which may be an advantage over HPLC.
- *Selecting the HPLC/CZE system*: Therefore, the selected system must be able to detect the hemoglobin variations as defined by the antenatal or population screening program and measure HbA2 and HbF accurately and precisely at these cut-offs.
- HPLC is appropriate as a confirming approach if CE is being used as a screening method, or a sickling test may be taken into consideration if sickle cell trait is suspected.
- Older methods are cellulose acetate paper electrophoresis, isoelectric focusing (IEF), alkali and acid gel electrophoresis, sephadex column-based estimation of HbA2 and Alkali denaturation for

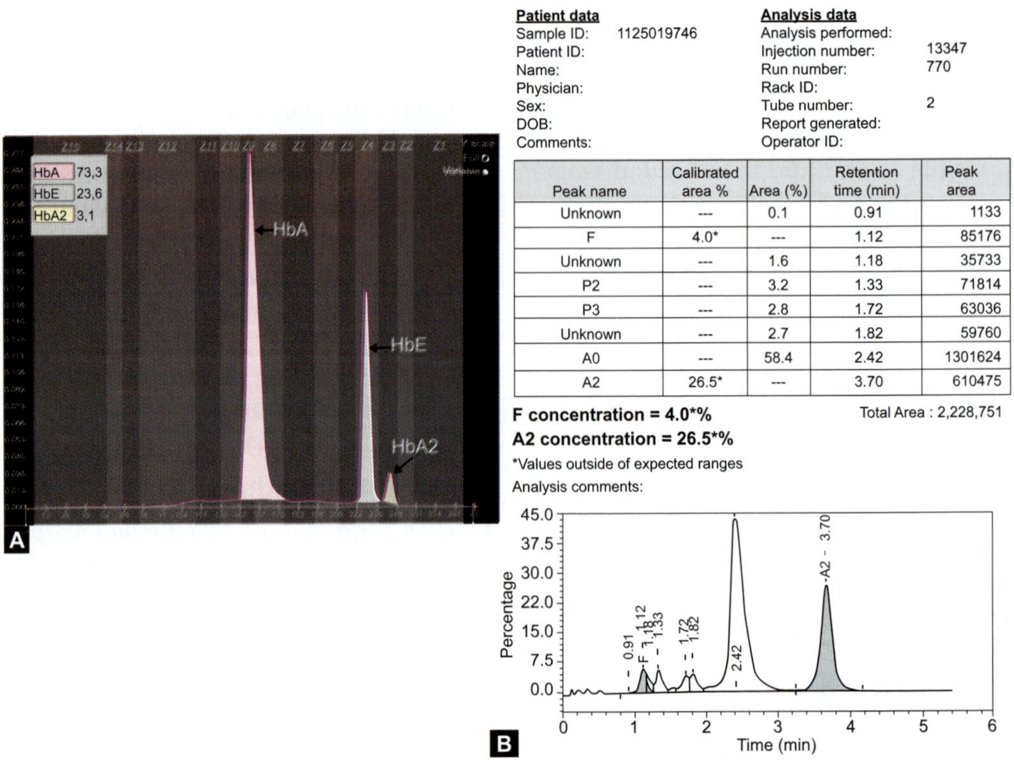

Patient data
Sample ID: 1125019746
Patient ID:
Name:
Physician:
Sex:
DOB:
Comments:

Analysis data
Analysis performed:
Injection number: 13347
Run number: 770
Rack ID:
Tube number: 2
Report generated:
Operator ID:

Peak name	Calibrated area %	Area (%)	Retention time (min)	Peak area
Unknown	---	0.1	0.91	1133
F	4.0*	---	1.12	85176
Unknown	---	1.6	1.18	35733
P2	---	3.2	1.33	71814
P3	---	2.8	1.72	63036
Unknown	---	2.7	1.82	59760
A0	---	58.4	2.42	1301624
A2	26.5*	---	3.70	610475

F concentration = 4.0*%
A2 concentration = 26.5*%
Total Area : 2,228,751
*Values outside of expected ranges
Analysis comments:

FIGS. 1A AND B: Cases of heterozygous for HbE/A. CZE showing separate peaks of HbA2 and Hb whereas, HPLC showing co-elution of HbE with HbA2.

HbF estimation are still being used in few centers. Densitometry is not recommended for estimation of HbA2 and HbF anymore.[1]

- *Cellulose acetate electrophoresis (CAE)*:
  - Using a cellulose acetate membrane for hemoglobin electrophoresis at a pH of 8.4 to 8.6 is an easy, dependable, and rapid technique. However, its usage is steadily declining in high-income nations and India due to the demand for handling large workloads efficiently. Despite this, it remains a practical approach in resource-limited settings and serves as a supplementary technique following HPLC as a second method to confirm rare types of abnormal Hb and in cases with fast moving bands on HPLC.
  - This method facilitates the preliminary identification of hemoglobins such as A, F, S/G/D, C/E/O-Arab, H, and several other less common variants. Differentiation between hemoglobins with similar migration patterns can be achieved using acid (agarose) gel electrophoresis, HPLC, or IEF. The issue of fast moving HbH in HPLC can be resolved by this test or by HbH bodies
- After electrophoresis/staining, scanning densitometry can be used to quantify variant hemoglobins, like HbS. However, it is not advised to use this method to quantify hemoglobin A2, as the precision is insufficient for diagnosing beta thalassemia trait.[13]
- *Sickling test*: Carrying out the sickling test is part of the diagnostic work up in patients suspected of having sickle cell syndrome. The test should be also carried out if there is an abnormal electrophoretic or chromatographic hemoglobin fraction in the position of HbS. It also helps to differentiate HbS from other variant hemoglobins like Hb Vellore, Hb Haaglanden and Hb Rush which elute in the S-window on HPLC and requires alkali gel electrophoresis and molecular studies for diagnosis **(Figs. 2A to C)**. A positive test is seen in both sickle cell trait and sickle cell disease. It is important to examine the preparation carefully as per the testing guidelines.
- *Detection of hemoglobin H bodies (HbH bodies)*:
  - When stained with supravital dyes like brilliant cresyl blue or new methylene blue, hemoglobin H bodies—intracellular deposits made of β4 tetramers—can be seen inside red blood cells.
  - These inclusions are particularly useful for confirming a diagnosis of Hb H disease, as they appear as golf-ball-like structures in approximately 5% of red blood cells after staining. Additionally, identifying HbH bodies can aid in the investigation of suspected acquired HbH disease or ATRX syndrome.
- *Quantification of HbF—issues with methods used*:
  - Quantification of HbF is indicated if HbF is raised beyond infancy.
  - A Keilhauer test can help distinguish between thalassemia major/TDT or intermedia/NTDT, suspected HPFH, suspected δβ thalassemia, and suspected bone marrow failure or neoplastic disorders such Diamond-Blackfan anemia and juvenile myelomonocytic leukemia. It shows pan cellular distribution of HbF in cases of HPFH and heterocellular staining in cases of δβ thalassemia. The results have to be interpreted along with the red cell indices and conformed only by DNA analysis.
  - The 2-min alkali denaturation test is suitable for the quantification of HbF levels <15% but significantly underestimates higher levels and is now rarely used.[14]

Peak name	Calibrated area (%)	Area (%)	Retention time (min)	Peak area
Unknown	---	0.1	1.00	1739
F	0.6	---	1.08	7959
Unknown	---	0.9	1.20	13730
P2	---	2.3	1.33	34449
P3	---	3.4	1.71	49977
A0	---	58.3	2.46	861492
A2	4.1*	---	3.65	64361
Unknown	---	30.1	4.57	444683

Total area: 1,478,391

F concentration = 0.6%
A2 concentration = 4.1*%

*Values outside of expected ranges

Analysis comments:

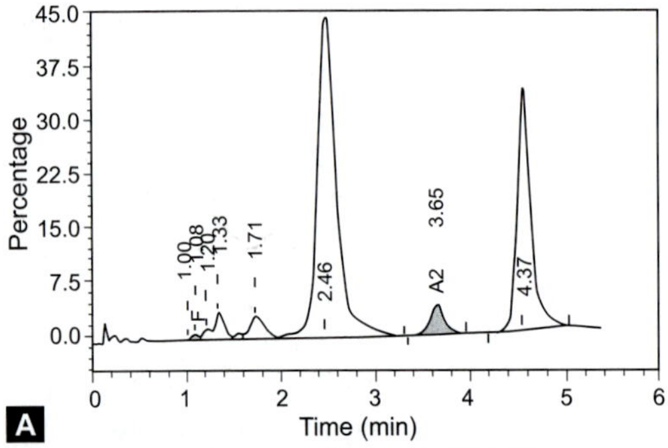

Peak name	Calibrated area (%)	Area (%)	Retention time (min)	Peak area
Unknown	---	0.1	0.99	1424
F	0.9	---	1.10	22969
Unknown	---	1.0	1.19	24691
P2	---	2.1	1.32	55138
P3	---	2.5	1.71	64447
A0	---	56.8	2.39	1464183
A2	2.8	---	3.66	73899
Unknown	---	33.8	4.36	871053

Total area: 2.577,805

F concentration = 0.9%
A2 concentration = 2.8*%

Analysis comments:

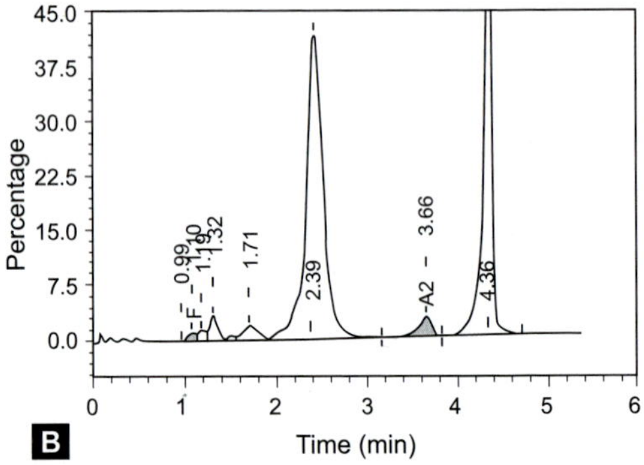

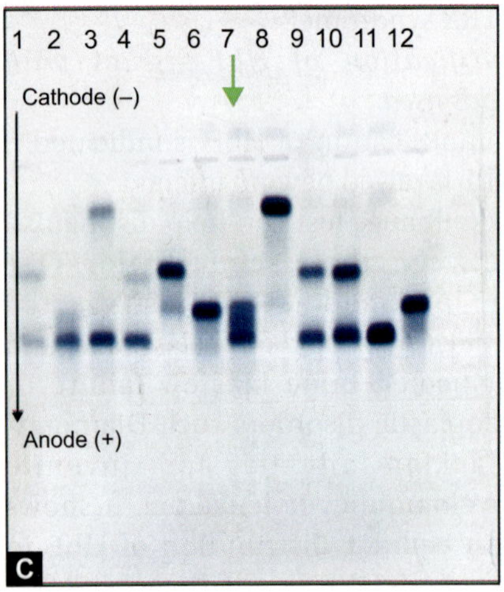

FIGS. 2A TO C: High performance liquid chromatogram (biorad variant II beta-thalassemia short program) of the patient with Hb Rush (HBB: c.304G>C); (A) an abnormal peak in the S-window comprising 30.1% with retention time of 4.57minutes. The peak has a broad base with a slant toward end, compared to the chromatogram of a sickle cell trait patient; (B) a peak in the S-window comprising 33.8% with retention time of 4.36 minutes, but the peak is sharp with a narrow base. (C) Alkali gel electrophoresis of the patient showing three bands (green arrow): One band in the HbA region and two distinct closely placed bands between HbF and HbA region. No band was seen in HbS/D/G region.

- The drawback of HPLC quantification is that it separates and hence excludes the adducted (post-translational) derivatives of Hb F, which might result in a notable underestimation at high concentrations. With CE, adducts of HbF are included in the estimate of HbF.[12]

GENERAL CONSIDERATIONS WHEN CHOOSING HPLC/CE SYSTEM

- The selected system should be able to estimate HbA2 and HbF accurately and precisely, as their recommended values have been used to act according to the National guidelines; for HbA2 cutoff of

≥3.5% for diagnosis pf β thalassemia carries in antenatal screening. For HbF two values have been set (≥5% and ≥10%, depending on the MCH)

- Laboratories should be aware of the integration in HPLC peaks which appear as shoulders on adjacent peaks and sloping baselines which are less reliable.
- Using a separate column or buffer solution for each test is necessary because using the same equipment or elution solution for several analytes (such as HbA2 and HbA1c) may affect the measurement of HbA2 and HbF. *This is an issue with D10 HPLC being used in small labs where it's used simultaneously for both tests.*[4]
- It is not advised to quantify HbA2 using CAE plus scanning densitometry; instead, CAE plus elution is suitable. A new diagnostic method based on microchip electrophoresis (Gazelle) is a point-of-care screening test providing identification and quantification of HbA2, HbF, HbS and HbA.[15] It has demonstrated 100% sensitivity and specificity in distinguishing β-thalassemia major/intermedia from healthy individuals and carriers, and 100% sensitivity with 98.3% specificity in identifying β-thalassemia trait in Indian settings.[16,17] Moreover, HbE can also be confirmed with high accuracy, making the system highly relevant for the Indian subcontinent, where HbS, β-thalassemia, and HbE constitute the majority of hemoglobinopathies. Given its affordability, portability, accuracy, and rapid turnaround time, microchip electrophoresis (Gazelle) is considered the preferred methodology for screening and confirmatory testing at community and primary healthcare facility levels, including subcenters, additional PHCs, PHCs, and CHCs.
- Controls should be performed on each batch, just like with any other hemoglobin analysis procedure. Variants are only tentatively identified, and confirmation should be obtained using complementing second-line techniques.
- Participation in external quality assessment should be promoted as advised by NABL and NQAS by Government of India, for satisfactory performance.
- A supplemental method suitable for the suspected anomaly should be used to confirm abnormal laboratory screening results.
- *Considerations for a standardized reporting*:
    - Sample date must be provided.
    - Transfusion history must be provided, including any in-utero blood transfusions.
    - If there is likely to be a delay in final reporting, an interim report must be informed to the clinician especially, in cases of sickle cell diseases.
    - The CBC parameters, red cell indices must be mentioned in the hemoglobinopathy report.
    - The results of a complimentary test (e.g., sickling test, Keilhauer test, and HbH inclusion test) should be included in the report.
    - Information about ethnicity, if available, should be part of the final report.

CONCLUSION

The implementation of standardized thalassemia testing guidelines in India marks a pivotal step toward reducing the burden of hemoglobinopathies through early detection, informed counseling, and timely intervention. These guidelines not only promote uniformity in diagnostic practices across diverse healthcare settings but also emphasize the importance of genetic literacy, community awareness, and ethical responsibility.

SUMMARY

- The diagnosis of heterozygous β thalassemia should be made based on the red blood cell indices and the HbA2 percentage.

- A diagnosis of heterozygous δβ thalassemia must be made because of the RBC indices (mainly MCH) and the HbF percentage.
- The diagnosis of α^0 thalassemia heterozygosity should be suspected based on the MCH and a normal or low hemoglobin A2 in a person of suitable family origin. The mother's DNA should be analyzed to confirm the diagnosis, and the biological father's DNA should be analyzed if the same diagnosis is suspected.
- In mothers with β thalassemia or HbE heterozygosity, the likelihood of co-existing α_0 thalassemia heterozygosity should be evaluated based on family origin. When the diagnosis would be important for reproductive decision-making, DNA analysis should be performed.
- The suspected presence of a significant variant of hemoglobin should be confirmed by a suitable alternative method.
- As there are approximately 1,800 genes associated with hemoglobinopathies the role of NGS is emerging for molecular screening and will be discussed in molecular diagnostic section
- Antenatal screening should be performed for thalassemia, sickle cell diseases and other clinically relevant hemoglobinopathies like, compound heterozygous states or homozygous states with thalassemia and sickle cell diseases
- Care must be taken for variants co-eluting with HbA2 like Hb Lepore, Hb D-Iran and HbE.
- Abnormal screening outcomes must be confirmed by a complementary method that is suitable for the likely abnormality.
- While using red cell indices in pregnant women we need to remember that the MCV increases by 3 fL and total RBC count decreases as part of normal physiology of pregnancy and the indices like Mentzer's are not good for screening.
- Testing should be performed on women who present for the first time late in pregnancy since the results will be useful for this and subsequent pregnancies and will allow the healthcare provider to provide genetic recommendations regarding future pregnancies.
- Partner screening in a high prevalence population for antenatal women partners, samples may be collected for early decision on prenatal diagnosis of homozygous or double heterozygous thalassemia after proper genetic counseling.

The National Health Mission Guidelines for hemoglobinopathies in India, clearly lays down the requisites for prenatal diagnosis and must be carried out in "at risk" couples after proper genetic counseling and written informed consent.

- Evaluation for hemoglobinopathies should be considered in all cases of unexplained microcytosis.
- For the phenotype of thalassemia intermedia, molecular analysis is still the gold standard for diagnosis, as they may have β^+ homozygosity or β^0 heterozygosity or double heterozygosity with α thalassemia, HbE or sickle trait **(Figs. 3 and 4)**.
- Thus, all cases for diagnosis need to be worked up for thalassemia syndromes e.g., HbE syndromes, HbE- β thalassemia, HbS- β thalassemia HbS- δβ thalassemia, Hbs-HPFH, etc., and family studies and molecular studies help in final diagnosis.
- The chosen system for screening and diagnosis of hemoglobinopathies should be able to measure HbA2 and HbF accurately and precisely, as their recommended values have been used to act according to the national guidelines; for HbA2 cutoff of ≥3.5% for diagnosis pf β thalassemia carries in antenatal

Peak name	Calibrated area (%)	Area (%)	Retention time (min)	Peak area
Unknown	---	0.4	0.87	5220
F	94.2*	---	1.21	1051725
A0	---	5.3	2.59	62397
A2	4.2*	---	3.69	55080

Total area: 1,174,422

F concentration = 94.2*%
A2 concentration = 4.2*%

*Values outside of expected ranges

Analysis comments:

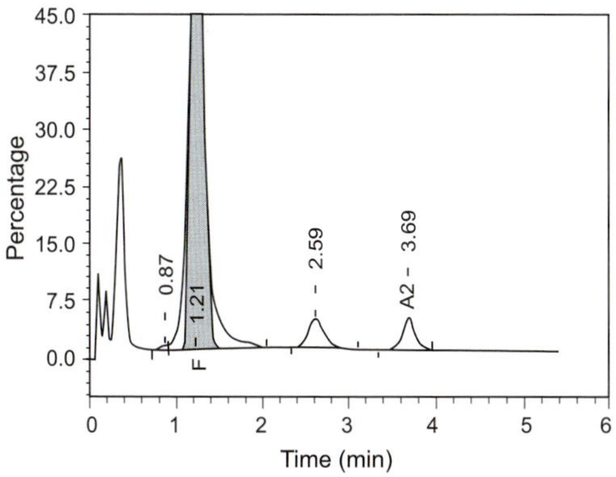

FIG. 3: Hb-HPLC showing prominent peaks of HbF (94.2%) and raised HbA2 (4.2%) in a case of compound heterozygous for HPFH with beta-thalassemia. RBC: 5.16 × 1012/L, Hb: 12.6 g/dL, MCV: 76 fL, MCH: 28 pg, MCHC: 34 g/dL, and RDW: 14% (biorad variant II beta-thalassemia short program).

Peak name	Calibrated area %	Area (%)	Retention time (min)	Peak area
Unknown	---	0.1	0.66	2047
P1	---	0.4	0.91	6210
F	48.2*	---	1.16	717549
P3	---	2.2	1.83	33936
A0	---	2.0	2.23	31346
Unknown	---	0.9	2.43	13430
A2	45.9*	---	3.71	728871

Total Area: 1,533,389

F concentration = 48.2*%
A2 concentration = 45.9*%

*Values outside of expected ranges

Analysis comments:

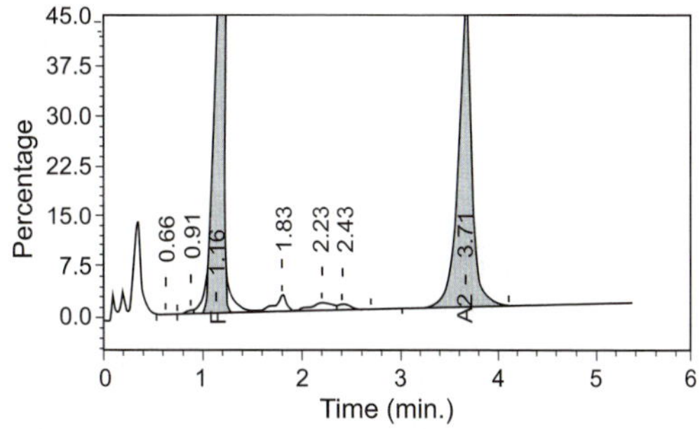

FIG. 4: Hb-HPLC showing prominent peaks of HbF (48.2%) and raised HbA2 (45.9%) in a case of compound heterozygous for HbE with beta thalassemia. RBC: 5.97 × 10/L, Hb: 9 g/dL, MCV: 62.7 fL, MCH: 19.1 pg and RDW: 19.5% (biorad variant II beta thalassemia short program).

screening. For HbF two values have been set (≥5% and ≥10%, depending on the MCH)

- Laboratories should be aware of the integration in HPLC peaks which appear as shoulders on adjacent peaks and sloping baselines which are less reliable.
- Participation in external quality assessment should be promoted as advised by NABL and NQAS by Government of India, for satisfactory performance.
- Abnormal screening outcomes must be confirmed by a complementary method that is suitable for the likely abnormality.

REFERENCES

1. Bain BJ, Bates I, Laffan MA. Dacie and Lewis Practical Haematology e-book. London: Elsevier Health Sciences; 2016.
2. Hoffmann JJ, Urrechaga E, Aguirre U. Discriminant indices for distinguishing thalassemia and iron deficiency in patients with microcytic anemia: A meta-analysis. Clin Chem Lab Med. 2015;53(12):1883-94.
3. Kotwal J, Saxena R, Choudhry VP, et al. Erythrocyte indices for discriminating thalassaemic and non-thalassaemic microcytosis in Indians. Natl Med J India. 1999;12(6):266-7.
4. Bain BJ, Daniel Y, Henthorn J, et al; BSH Committee. Significant haemoglobinopathies: A guideline for screening and diagnosis: A British Society for Haematology Guideline: A British Society

for Haematology Guideline. Br J Haematol. 2023;201(6):1047-65.
5. Ministry of Health and Family Welfare, Government of India. NHM Guidelines for Prevention and Control of Hemoglobinopathies in India. Chapter: Prenatal Diagnosis—Preventing the Birth of an Affected Child of "At Risk Couple". India: Ministry of Health and Family Welfare; 2021. pp. 57-9.
6. Galanello R, Barrela R Ideo A, et al. Genotype of subjects with borderline HbA2: implications of beta- thalassemia carrier screening. Am J H ematol. 1994;46:79-81.
7. Urrechaga E, Borque L, Escanero JF. Erythrocyte and reticulocyte parameters in iron deficiency and thalassemia. J Clin Lab Anal. 2011;25(3):223-8.
8. Colah R, Thomas M, Mayekar P. Assessing the impact of screening and counselling high school children for beta-thalassaemia in India. J Med Screen. 2007;14(3):158.
9. Cappellini MD, Farmakis D, Porter J, et al. Guidelines for the Management of Transfusion-Dependent Thalassaemia, 4th ed. Nicosia, Cyprus: Thalassaemia International Federation; 2021.
10. Ryan K, Bain BJ, Worthington D, et al. Streetly a; British Committee for Standards in Haematology. Significant haemoglobinopathies: guidelines for screening and diagnosis. Br J Haematol. 2010;149(1):35-49.
11. Wild BJ, Stephens AD. The use of automated HPLC to detect and quantitate haemoglobins. Clin Lab Haematol. 1997;19(3):171-6.
12. Shihabi ZK, Hinsdale ME, Daugherty HK, Jr. Hemoglobin A2 quantification by capillary zone electrophoresis. Electrophoresis. 2000;21:749-52.
13. Bain BJ, Amos RJ, Bareford D, Chapman C, et al. The laboratory diagnosis of haemoglobinopathies. Br J Haematol. 1998;101(4):783-92.
14. Stephens AD, Angastiniotis M, Baysal E, et al. ICSH recommendations for the measurement of Haemoglobin F. Int J Lab Hematol. 2012;34: 14-20.
15. Canatan D, Delibaş S, Altunsoy E, et al. A New Diagnostic Method for Premarital Screening of Thalassemia and Hemoglobinopathies: Microchip Electrophoresis (Gazelle) Method. Blood. 2024;144:1094.
16. Ran AN, Avanaki A, Thota P, et al. Point-of-Care Diagnostic Test for Beta-Thalassemia. Biosensors. 2024;14(2):83.
17. Jain A, Jena RK, Dolai TK, et al. Exploring Advances in Point-of-Care Diagnosis: Microchip Electrophoresis for Hemoglobinopathy Detection in Indian Populations. Blood. 2024;144(Supplement 1):3621.

3

CHAPTER

Thalassemia Syndromes: Clinical Features

Ashish Dixit

INTRODUCTION

Thalassemia syndromes are hereditary disorders characterized by reduced or absent synthesis of beta or alpha globin chains, leading to decreased hemoglobin in red blood cells and resulting in anemia. Clinically, thalassemia can be categorized into transfusion-dependent thalassemia (TDT or thalassemia major), nontransfusion-dependent thalassemia (NTDT or thalassemia intermedia), and thalassemia minor. The clinical phenotypes of homozygous or compound heterozygous beta-thalassemia manifest as thalassemia major and intermedia, with considerable variability in the phenotypic spectrum and severity, particularly in HbE/beta-thalassemia. **Figure 1** describes the transfusion requirements across thalassemia spectrum. TDT patients usually present within the first 2 years of life and require regular red cell transfusions for survival, whereas NTDT patients have a later onset and typically do not need frequent transfusions. Heterozygous thalassemia often results in a silent carrier state. The number of transfusions in the preceding 6 months

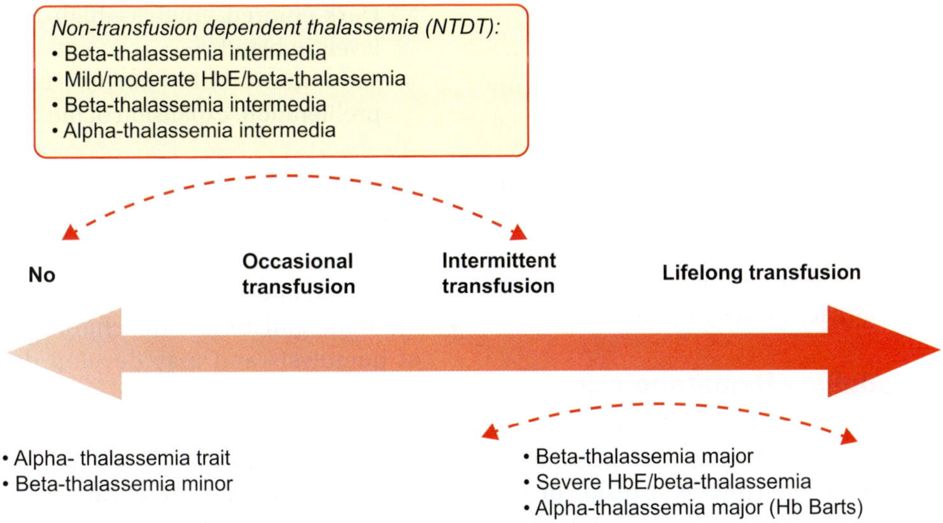

FIG. 1: Transfusion requirements in various phenotypes of thalassemia.

can serve as a rough guide to distinguish TDT from NTDT, with fewer than six units suggesting NTDT. However, this classification should be reassessed dynamically, as NTDT patients may progress to TDT over time, while some TDT patients may transition to NTDT following appropriate interventions.

TRANSFUSION-DEPENDENT THALASSEMIA (THALASSEMIA MAJOR)

- Between 6 and 24 months is when TDT (thalassemia major) first manifests clinically.
- Infants affected become more pale and do not thrive.
- Common symptoms are feeding problems, irritability and abdominal distension due to splenomegaly and liver enlargement.
- Clinical manifestations of the TDT (thalassemia major) are due to:
  - Severe anemia
  - Extramedullary hematopoiesis
  - Complications of hemolysis
  - Iron overload

Anemia

- The quantity of globin chains generated and the number of functional globin chains are correlated with the prevalence and severity of anemia.
- Anemia manifestations depend on severity of anemia and can range from easy fatigue, dizziness, dyspnea on exertion, palpitations and sometimes frank cardiac failure symptoms.

Extramedullary Hematopoiesis

- Inefficient erythropoiesis is the term used to describe inefficient RBC generation in the bone marrow as a result of the loss of developing RBC precursors. As a consequence, skeletal deformities are caused by erythropoiesis developing outside of the bone marrow.
- *Skeletal changes include*:
  - Abnormalities of long bones of the legs
  - Craniofacial deformities
  - Frontal bossing
  - Malar prominence
  - Depressed nasal bridge
  - Maxillary hypertrophy leading to expose the upper teeth
- *Facial features and their causes*:
  - *Dental malocclusion*: Maxillary prominence and mandibular atrophy
  - *Lateral orbital displacement*: Overgrowth of marrow in the maxillary bone
  - Chipmunk features include frontal bossing, saddle nose, and malar prominence.
  - Paranasal sinus pneumatization and marrow hyperplasia in the frontal, temporal, and facial bones
- *Oral manifestations and their causes*:
  - Poor oral hygiene, lower salivary phosphorus and IgA levels, and a high caries index
  - Atrophic glossitis, and mucosal pallor
  - Dark-colored gingiva—high ferritin levels in blood
  - Thin mandibular cortex—marrow proliferation, expansion of medulla

Complications of Hemolysis

- Jaundice is commonly seen in patients with both TDT and NTDT (thalassemia major and intermedia)
- Pigment gallstones are characteristic of hemolysis and may develop during childhood itself
- Chronic hemolysis, extramedullary hematopoiesis in the liver and spleen, and hepatic iron accumulation can all lead to hepatosplenomegaly.

Complications of Iron Overload (Discussed in Detail in Other Relevant Chapters)

- As people age, the clinical phenotype of those with severe thalassemia (TDT) may become dominated by clinical signs of iron overload.
- Heart failure is the primary clinical issue that can cause premature death.
- Significant issues also arise from endocrine imbalances, specifically hypogonadism, low growth hormone, hypothyroidism, and diabetes mellitus.
- Liver iron deposition can be significant, although unless iron overload is quite severe, functional impairments are often minor.

Nontransfusion-dependent Thalassemia (Thalassemia Intermedia)

- Patients with NTDT show a markedly heterogeneous clinical picture.
- By definition, patients with NTDT do not require lifelong regular transfusion for survival. Transfusions may be occasionally required or frequently required in certain clinical settings for a short period of time.
- All the symptoms related to extramedullary hematopoiesis get more prominent in thalassemia intermedia due to compensation by erythroid hyperactivity.
- Principle symptoms are pallor, jaundice, cholelithiasis, hepatosplenomegaly, moderate to severe skeletal changes, leg ulcers, extramedullary masses of hyperplastic erythroid marrow, a tendency to develop osteopenia and osteoporosis
- Thrombotic complications may be seen resulting from a hypercoagulable state because of the lipid membrane composition of the abnormal red blood cells (particularly in splenectomized patients).
- Iron overload occurs mainly from increased intestinal absorption of iron caused by ineffective erythropoiesis.
- Leg ulcers may develop in NTDT (thalassemia intermedia). Underlying factors include a combination of chronic anemia, tissue damage, iron overload, venous stasis, bone deformities and local trauma.

THALASSEMIA MINOR

- Individuals with one mutated globin gene are thalassemia carriers or minor
- Depending on the severity of the mutation, some patients may still have mild anemia.
- Mild unconjugated jaundice is not uncommon in thalassemia minor
- Early onset pigment gallstones may also be seen.
- No other manifestations related to iron overload or extramedullary erythropoiesis are seen.

CONCLUSION

Thalassemia syndromes represent inherited disorders of globin synthesis with varying clinical severity. TDT presents early with severe anemia and iron overload-related complications, while NTDT shows variable anemia, extramedullary hematopoiesis, and gradual iron accumulation. Thalassemia minor remains largely asymptomatic with mild anemia. Recognizing the clinical spectrum is crucial for timely diagnosis, appropriate transfusion support, and prevention of complications. Regular monitoring and individualized management are essential to improve survival and quality of life in affected patients.

SUMMARY

- Thalassemia syndromes include TDT, NTDT and thalassemia minor, classified by severity and transfusion dependence.

- TDT (thalassemia major) presents in infancy with severe anemia, requiring lifelong transfusions, while NTDT (thalassemia intermedia) has variable severity.
- Complications include skeletal deformities, extramedullary hematopoiesis, jaundice, and hepatosplenomegaly.
- Iron overload from transfusions leads to endocrine dysfunction, cardiac failure, and liver fibrosis.
- Thalassemia minor is usually asymptomatic with mild anemia and no major complications.

SUGGESTED READINGS

1. Taher AT, Musallam KM, Cappellini MD. β-Thalassemias. N Engl J Med. 2021;384(8):727-43.
2. Cappellini MD, Farmakis D, Porter J, et al. Guidelines for the Management of Transfusion-Dependent Thalassaemia, 4th edition, Version 2.0. Nicosia, Cyprus: Thalassaemia International Federation; 2021.
3. Taher AT, Musallam KM, Cappellini MD. Guidelines for the Management of Non-Transfusion-Dependent β-Thalassaemia, 3rd edition. Nicosia, Cyprus: Thalassaemia International Federation; 2023.
4. Taher AT, Saliba AN, Taher A, et al. Clinical Complications and Their Management. Blood Rev. 2018;32(2):107-22.
5. Sadiq IZ, Abubakar FS, Usman HS, et al. Thalassemia: Pathophysiology, Diagnosis, and Advances in Treatment. Thalass Rep. 2024;14(4): 81-102.
6. Musallam KM, Rivella S, Vichinsky E, et al. Non-transfusion-dependent thalassemias. Haematologica. 2013;98(6):833-44.

Chapter 4

Prevention and Control of Thalassemia

Maitreyee Bhattacharyya

INTRODUCTION

Thalassemia and structural variants of hemoglobins like sickle cell anemia are the most common single gene disorders worldwide. Around 300,000 to 400,000 babies with severe hemoglobin disorder are born each year.[1] The majority of babies being born in middle and low income countries.[2]

Thalassemias and sickle cell disease (SCD) are major public health problems in India. The prevalence of beta thalassemia carriers is 3–4% on average but some areas has prevalence as high as 15–17%.[3,4] It is expected that there would be around 100,000 patients with a beta thalassemia and around 150,000 cases of SCD.[5,6] However, there is no National Registry so difficult to get the exact number.

It has been suggested that around 32,400 babies are expected to be born each year with hemoglobin disorders.[7,8] Population screening for thalassemia carriers and prevention of birth of affected children is the need of the day.

INHERITANCE

Thalassemia and other hemoglobinopathies are mostly an autosomal recessive disorder. When one of the parents is carrier and other normal there is 50% chance that the offspring will be carrier and 50% normal **(Flowchart 1)**. When both the parents are carriers there is a 25% chance of having a thalassemia affected baby, 50% thalassemia carrier and 25% normal. This is applicable for each pregnancy **(Flowchart 2)**.

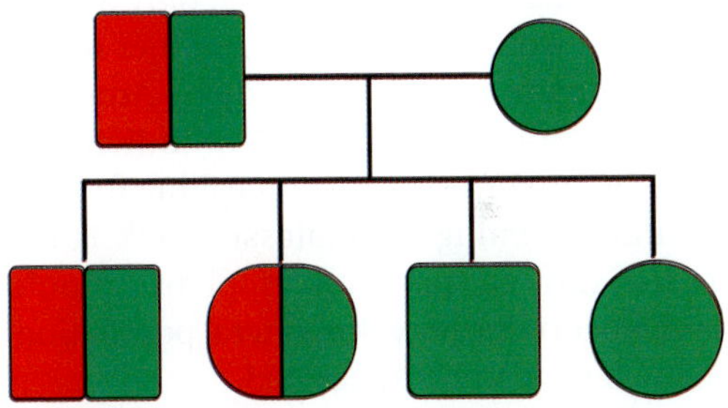

FLOWCHART 1: One parent is thalassemia carrier and other normal.

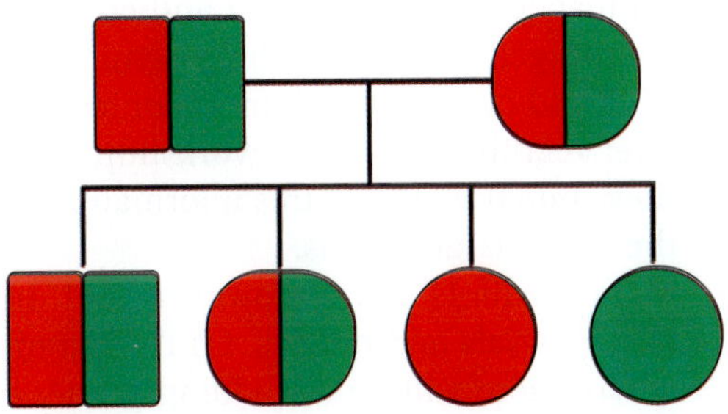

FLOWCHART 2: Both the parents are thalassemia carrier.

CONTROL PROGRAM

It consists of four main pillars:

1. Awareness generation
2. Screening of population

3. Prenatal diagnosis
4. Adequate care of the affected child.

Awareness Generation

Over the past few decades various institutions in India as well as social organizations and NGOs have been conducting awareness programs. Yet, awareness about thalassemia is very poor all over India. A study done by Srivastava JK et al. showed that in the medium to low socioeconomic and educational background targeted population in South 24 Parganas district in West Bengal only 37.93% heard the word thalassemia.[9] Another recent questionnaire based KAP study by Aroras in north India found that >50% of individuals from the urban area were not willing for pre-marital screening for thalassemia.[10] These studies showed that more emphasis should be given on educating the general population. Following measures suggested.

- Inclusion of thalassemia, SCD, and other hemoglobinopathies information in textbooks of high schoolchildren.[11]
- All teachers of high school and colleges should get training on thalassemia and SCD and other hemoglobinopathies just after recruitment (1 day workshop) and they should percolate this information to the students/guardians.
- Mass media is a very powerful tool. In all TV serials and movies, OTT program where there will be a wedding scene, a subtitle should scroll in local language "get your blood tested before marriage" (this is like anti-smoking campaign).[12]
- A short clip on beta-thalassemia and SCD by a leading film personality during prime time television programs shown over a period of time would have a significant impact on the population at large.[12]
- All advertisement related to wedding materials should also bear this caption
- Matrimonial page in all the newspapers should have this message in every page
- Websites for matrimony also should mention this.
- To get a certificate to work as marriage register training on thalassemia should be must
- All marriage registration offices should display message about thalassemia
- All Priests, Moulavi and Fathers in the charge should be trained to motivate persons to check thalassemia carrier status before marriage
- Display should be there in all hospitals and health centers about information of thalassemia and its prevention (like previously done for birth control).
- ASHA workers should be trained in this knowledge so that they will educate villagers during their home visit.
- The most important message to be given is that "Thalassemia carriers are absolutely healthy. If a carrier marries another carrier then there is a chance of having a thalassemia affected child. If two carriers can get married, they should take help of prenatal diagnosis to avoid birth of thalassemia affected children. However if a carrier marries a noncarrier there is no risk of thalassemia affected child "
- ASHA workers usually organize group discussion on various health issues. Thalassemia and sickle cell anemia should be included in these and local public representative should be requested to be present.
- Local NGOs should be encouraged to take part in awareness generation and screening.[2]

Screening of Population

Screening of population, identification of carriers and prevention of marriage between two carriers are the cornerstones of thalassemia control. India is a large country with a population of around 133 crore. Neither its possible nor its required to screen the whole population. Screening should be voluntary where the participants make an informed choice and once they undergo screening, the next step to follow should be counseling, however this is not always the case.

Whom to Screen?

Screening of population of reproductive age group 15–45 years of age.

- *High school children*:[13,14] Class IX students of each school every year need to be considered. This will ultimately lead to screening of all students who passed out of that school. The program should be chalked out along with the education department of the state. District school inspectors should also undergo training and should be a part of the program.
- During admission in College[15,16] carrier screening status of the students may be checked, if it's not there it can be done on the spot.
- Premarital group[17-19] coming voluntarily for screening or sent by ASHA workers. Premarital screening is affected by socio-cultural barriers where parents often do not wish to reveal the carrier status of their children premaritally for fear of difficulty in marriage prospects. This is specially applicable for girls. So in premarital screening boys should be screened first, if the boy is normal, the girl may not be screened.
- Thalassemia screening can be done of the patients attending adolescent clinics of all government hospitals and medical colleges
    - *Postmarital preconceptional screening*: ASHA workers should take the initiative in rural areas. Obstetricians should make it compulsory for the couples attending their clinic for pre-conception checkup and advice.
    - *Antenatal mothers*: Pregnant women attending antenatal clinic should be screened during their first visit.[20,21] This should be irrespective of their parity and gestational age. Husbands of detected carrier women should be screened. If both of them are carriers, pre-natal diagnosis should be advised.
- *Neonatal screening*: In areas where sickle cell prevalence is high, neonatal screening should be mandatory.[22,23]
- *Targeted screening*: The screening programs undertaken till date in different regions have shown that many ethnic groups have much higher prevalence rates than the average ranging from 4 to 17% **(Table 1)**.[2-5,24-27] Thus, targeted screening in such high-risk groups is acceptable and should be undertaken.
- *Extended family screening*:[28,29] Once a person is detected to be thalassemia carrier, siblings and other members of the reproductive age group should be screened.
- Reproductive age group population attending blood donation camp can be screened taking help of transfusion medicine/blood bank.

Who will Screen?

- All Medical Colleges and district hospitals should have a team designated for thalassemia. This should comprise one medical officer, two technicians, one counselor. They will organize regular camps in schools, colleges and antenatal clinics.

TABLE 1: Communities with high prevalence of beta-thalassemia.[2]

Communities	Prevalence of thalassaemia
Sindhis, Lohans, Bhanushalis, Vellalas	8–17%
Vasava, Chaudhry, Kokana tribes,	12–15%
Aroras, Khatris, Jaths	6–10%
Prajapatis, Banias, Jains, Mayavanshis	6–8%
Bhuyan, Pik, Dudh Kharia tribes, Rohit tribes	6–8%
Kayastha, Mandols	5–9%
Menons, Shiyas, Fakirs	5–7%
Neobuddhists, Mahars	4–6%

- *Subdivisional hospitals/PHC/SHC*:
  - One designated technician for thalassemia screening
  - All ASHA workers should be trained for thalassemia counseling.

How to Screen?

Pretest counseling: Person to be screened should be informed about the inheritance, disease manifestations and necessity of screening. Informed consent should be taken prior to screening.

In case of camps a short presentation to be given before the mass. This presentation should be a government approved fixed one, and can be downloaded from government portals.

Point of care testing should be done for all antenatal mothers/premarital person/ preconceptional persons sent by ASHA worker[30] to the PHC/subcenter.

Methods of Testing

- PHC/SHC/subdivisional hospitals
- Point-of-care testing approved by government of India

Screening at District Hospitals/ Medical Colleges

- *Method*: Two cc of blood to be collected in EDTA vial.
- Complete hemogram
- Samples with MCV < 85 to be run for HPLC

Data Recording

Data regarding the person screened to be entered into the software by the screening person. Software should include minimal data to be user friendly.

- Age
- Sex
- Address
- Mobile No
- Aadhaar No
- Test ID—no/date/District/State
- Religion
- Caste
- Premarital/preconception/antenatal/ others
- Hb
- RBC
- MCV
- MCH
- HPLC

POSTSCREENING COUNSELING

- Carriers should undergo counseling before getting the report.
- Maintain confidentiality of the detected carriers wherever, screening for carriers is carried out.
- Any person who detected to have thalassemia or SCD during screening should be sent to the nearest thalassemia center for proper treatment.

Steps of Neonatal Screening

Informed consent: An explanatory leaflet detailing the purpose, process and outcomes of newborn screening for sickle cell conditions must be provided to the parent(s) prior to screening. The purpose of screening should be explained by ANM or staff nurse during pregnancy and then again before taking the test.

Newborn sample: The same dried blood spot card is used for sickle screening as for the other newborn screening programs. For the complete and proper processing of the specimen, four good quality spots are required.

Report Format

Report format is shown in **Figure 1**.

Data Recording

- Most important for future plans or modification of existing plans.
- There should be a portal for thalassemia where two different software, one for

Name Age Sex
Aadhaar No. Mobile No.
Sample ID Date of collection Date of test

Hemogram
Hb
RBC
MCV
MCH
HPLC
HbA2 HbF HbA HbS HbD Others

Impression
Signature

FIG. 1: Report format.

population screening and another for thalassemia patients to be maintained.

- ASHA worker/data entry operators/ treating physician/will enter data of screening and patients data.
- Patients' data recording will be dynamic and should be updated from time to time.
- It should be mandatory for private practitioner/private lab to send the data of carrier or cases detected every month to the government authorities

Prevention Program

- *Primary level-ASHA, Ayushman Bharat Arogya Mandir, CHC, PHC, UPHC*
    - Asha workers will sensitize village population, arrange premarital screening
    - All pregnant ladies attending ANC will be tested for thalassemia carrier status irrespective of their gestational age and parity. Husbands of carrier mothers to be counseled for screening. If both husband and wife are carriers, the couple will be sent to the nearest medical college for prenatal diagnosis.
    - Government approved point of care testing should be done
    - Neonatal screening in areas of high prevalence of SCD. Dry blood spot to be collected and sent for testing.
- *Secondary level:* District hospitals—
    - Dedicated Medical Officer, Nurses, counselor and Data Entry Officer will be there in each district hospital
    - They will arrange for antenatal screening, all pregnant ladies irrespective of their gestational age and parity. Husbands of carrier mother to be tested and if both of them are carrier, couple to be sent to tertiary level for prenatal diagnosis
    - Involvement of obstetrician for antenatal screening/prenatal diagnosis
    - Obstetrician of district hospital will collect CVS/amniotic fluid sample
    - District hospital team will organize camps in school, colleges, blood donation camps
    - Run thalassemia clinic once in a week
    - Run day care center in 6 days/week
    - Will organize training of peripheral unit staffs/other nonmedical persons–marriage register, school teachers, etc.
    - *Equipment*: Cell counter, HPLC/ capillary electrophoresis machine, ELISA for Ferritin
    - Linkage of districts hospitals with apex centers will be established
    - Telemedicine to be used to discuss difficult cases with the center of excellence or referred for sequencing or additional tests if not available.
- *Tertiary level:* All medical colleges—
    - Dedicated Medical Officer, Nurses, counselor and Data Entry Officer will be there in each district hospital
    - They will arrange for antenatal screening, all pregnant ladies irrespective of their gestational age and parity. Husbands of carrier mother to be tested and if both of them are carrier, couple to be sent to tertiary level for prenatal diagnosis
    - Will organize camps in school, colleges, blood donation camps

- Run thalassemia clinic once in a week
- Run day care center in 6 days/week
- Will organize training of staffs of district hospitals
- *Equipment*: Cell counter, HPLC machine, ELISA for Ferritin
- Couple requiring prenatal diagnosis to be counseled properly and blood samples to be sent to higher centers for detection of mutation
- At least two obstetricians of each medical college to be trained for CVS. Any couple requiring prenatal diagnosis, CVS to be done and tissue to be sent to the higher centers

- *State level:* Regional Center of Excellence (Medical Colleges) at least 2 in each state it may be increased depending on the size of the state.
    - The center of excellence should be well dispersed throughout the state.
    - *Facilities*:
        - Manpower: Hematologist 1.MO 2, NS4, technician 4, counselor 4, molecular biologist 2, DEO 2
        - Equipment: Cell counter, HPLC machine, ELISA machine, PCR and gel dock, sangers sequencer, computer, printer
        - A blood bank facility with tertiary care capacity. Should have ability to do extended blood grouping and detection and typing of alloantibodies.
        - Facilities for providing HLA typing-at least low/intermediate resolution molecular HLA typing.
        - Center should have the capability to comprehensively evaluate and monitor cardiac and endocrine function in the patients including a MRIT2* facility.
        - Transcranial Doppler facility should be made available at every COE to annually screen children with sickle cell anemia from 2 to 16 years of age.
    - *Work schedule*: Outreach camp, antenatal camp, prenatal diagnosis, thalassemia clinic, day care, molecular testing as and when required.
    - Setting up centers for BMT for thalassemia patients
    - It should be directly or indirectly involved in conducting and supervising screening programs in the region that it oversees.
    - Should be actively involved in research activities
    - The designated COE should have active staff and facilities to maintain comprehensive data of all cases and carriers within the region they oversee

TRAINING OF THE STAFF AT DIFFERENT LEVELS

The staff employed in the project at various levels should be trained and sensitized in the activities to be performed by them through special training programs organized.

Modular training with hands on training should cover the following skills:

- Genetic counseling (for all staff)
- Performance of laboratory tests for carrier screening and diagnosis of hemoglobinopathies, (for laboratory technicians)
- Interpretation of laboratory tests and preparation of various reports (for pathologists and hematologists)
- Obstetrical procedures for obtaining fetal tissue like amniocentesis and chorionic villus sampling (for obstetricians, minimum 2 weeks)
- Molecular biology techniques for identification of molecular mutations and for prenatal diagnosis (for scientists, 2 weeks).
- Training for treatment of patients with thalassemia major, and SCD and taking care of the various complications (for physicians and pediatricians)

- Training in blood bank practices (for blood bank technician and medical officer

Monitoring

Monitoring and necessary modification of the program will be done by expert/ administrative committee at district/state/ national level

- *District administrative committee*:
  - Faculty from two medical colleges
  - Molecular biologist (if any)
  - Obstetrician designated for prenatal diagnosis
  - District school inspector
  - CMOH
  - Members of NGO2
- *State expert/administrative committee*:
  - At least two hematologist
  - One molecular biologist
  - One counselor
  - Member from at least 3 NGOs
  - Program officer (government administrative)
  - Software person (for analyzing collected data)
  - At least five public representatives
  - MD-NHM
  - DHS/DME
  - Health secretary
  - Education—secretary
- *National expert/administrative committee*:
  - At least two experts from each state
  - Health secretary
  - MD-NHM
  - Education secretary
  - Public representative
  - Members of NGO
  - Will monitor the program and take necessary action
  - Meet quarterly to analyze progress, identify lope holes
  - Sustained Advocacy measures to inform the population of the burden of disease and to build support for making available resources for its prevention and management of hemoglobinopathies.
  - Interact with the policy makers Convergence with linked ministries and departments (e.g., Ministry of Human Resource Development, Women and Child Development and Ministry of Social Justice and empowerment, Ministry of Tribal Affairs) at the national and state level to raise awareness and garner support for the program.
  - Engage with patient/parent's organizations and NGOs in the implementation of the national policy.
  - Prepare IEC material that is easily understood, informative and useful, and translate it into various regional languages.
  - Engage prominent spokes persons to reinforce the messages

CONCLUSION

India is a country which shares major burden of world thalassemia patients. It is felt that unless a major thrust is provided to the control programme, the ultimate goal of reducing the number of thalassemics born in India cannot be achieved satisfactorily in this decade.

In a country like India where limited knowledge of the hemoglobin disorders exists, doctors, nurses, and social workers needs to be trained in the basic diagnosis and management of the hemoglobin disorders. There is a need to increase the number of centers in India able to perform awareness generation, screening, and diagnosis.

SUMMARY

- *Epidemiological burden*: Thalassemia and SCD are among the most common single-gene disorders globally, with India contributing significantly to the disease burden—approximately 100,000 β-thalassemia and 150,000 SCD patients.
- *Core pillars of control program*: The national control strategy is built on four

pillars—awareness generation, population screening, prenatal diagnosis, and comprehensive care for affected individuals.

- *Awareness generation measures*:
  - Inclusion of thalassemia education in school curricula
  - Training programs for teachers and ASHA workers
  - Mass media campaigns with marriage-related health messages (e.g., "get your blood tested before marriage")
  - Engagement of NGOs, religious leaders, and public representatives for community education
- *Screening strategy*: Voluntary, informed screening of reproductive age group (15–45 years) is prioritized. Target groups include school and college students, premarital and antenatal couples, and high-prevalence communities.
- *Screening implementation*:
  - *Primary level*: PHCs and subcenters use *point-of-care testing*
  - *Secondary level*: District hospitals conduct HPLC-based testing
  - *Tertiary level*: Medical colleges and Centers of Excellence perform confirmatory tests and prenatal diagnostics
- *High-risk communities*: Certain ethnic groups show higher carrier prevalence (6–17%), e.g., Sindhis, Aroras, Kayasthas, Vellalas, Bhuyan and Kharia tribes. Targeted and extended family screening is strongly recommended.
- *Prenatal and neonatal screening*:
  - *Prenatal*: All antenatal women should be screened at first visit; if both partners are carriers, prenatal diagnosis (CVS/amniocentesis) is advised.
  - *Neonatal*: Dried blood spot testing for newborns in sickle cell-endemic regions.
- *Data management and reporting*: A national digital registry is essential for both carriers and patients. All screening data should be uploaded to a government portal, with private labs mandated to report cases monthly.
- *Three-tier implementation structure*:
  - *Primary level*: ASHA-driven community sensitization and screening.
  - *Secondary level*: District hospitals conduct screening, counseling, and weekly thalassemia clinics.
  - *Tertiary level*: Medical colleges/COEs provide prenatal diagnosis, molecular testing, and training of staff.
- *Training and capacity building*: Structured modular training for all cadres—ASHAs, laboratory technicians, obstetricians, hematologists, and counselors—covering genetic counseling, lab techniques, prenatal diagnostics, and patient management.
- *Monitoring and governance*: Multitiered committees (district, state, national) comprising hematologists, obstetricians, NGOs, and administrators will *review* program progress quarterly, modify strategies, and ensure inter-ministerial convergence.

REFERENCES

1. Williams TN, Weatherall DJ. World distribution, population genetics and health burden of the hemoglobinopathies. Cold Spring Harb Prospects Med. 2012;2:a011692
2. Cao A, Kan YW. The prevention of thalassemia. Cold Spring Harb Perspect Med. 2013;3:a011775
3. Madan N, Sharma S, Sood SK, et al. Frequency of b thalassemia trait and other hemoglobinopathies in northern and western India. Indian J Hum Genet. 2010;16:16-25.
4. Colah RB, Gorakshakar AC. Control of thalassemia in India. Thal Reports. 2014;4:1955.

5. Colah R, Mukherjee M, Ghosh K. Sickle cell disease in India. Curr Opin Hematol. 2014;21:215-23.
6. Verma IC, Saxena R, Kohli S. Past, present and future scenario of thalassemic care and control in India. Indian J Med Res. 2011;134:507-21.
7. Christianson A, Howson CP, Modell B. March of Dimes global report on birth Defects: the hidden toll of dying and disabled children. White Plains, New York: March of Dimes Birth Defects Foundation; 2006.
8. Grow K, Vashist M, Abrol P, et al. βthalassemia in India: current status and challenges ahead. Int J Pharm Pharm Sci. 2014;6:28-33.
9. Shrivastava JK, Sinha N, Behera SK, et al. Knowledge, attitude and practice study of β thalassemia in rural Bengal. Genet Clin. 2011;4:13-5.
10. Chawla S, Singh RK, Lakkakula B, et al. Attitudes and beliefs among high and low risk population groups towards b thalassemia prevention: across sectional descriptive study from India. J Community Genet. 2017;8:159-66.
11. Cao A, Kan YW. The prevention of thalassemia. Cold Spring Harb Perspect Med. 2013;3:a011775
12. Chandy M. Developing a national thalassemia control programme for India. In: Ghosh K, Colah R (Eds). Control and management of thalassemia and other hemoglobinopathies in the Indian subcontinent-synoptic views. Mumbai: National Institute of Immunohaematology; 2008. pp. 46-9.
13. Ragba SM, Elrahimb MA, El Fotoha WMA, et al. Ibrahimc Screening of β-thalassemia carriers in high school students in Shebin El-Kom, Menoufia Governorate. Menoufia Med J. 2021;34(1): 237-42.
14. Colah R, Thomas M, Mayekar P. Assessing the impact of screening and counselling high school children for beta-thalassaemia in India. J Med Screen. 2007;14(3):158.
15. Rishmitha, Badagabettu S, Archana MV et al. Awareness on thalassemia and opinion of carrier screening among young women from selected undergraduate colleges of UDUPI district. Clin Epidemiol Glob Health. 2022;14:100978.
16. Datar S, Poflee S. Premarital screening of college students for carrier detection in thalassemia and sickle cell disease: need of the hour. Int J Med Sci Public Health. 2015;4(3):1
17. Hashemizadeh H, Noori R. Premarital Screening of Beta Thalassemia Minor in north-east of Iran Iran J Ped Hematol Oncol. 2013;3(1):210-5.
18. Hussain Z. Pre-Marital Screening for Thalassaemia–Legal, Social and Technical Obstacles. National J Health Sci. 2018;3(2):33-3.
19. Suresh H, Jamil S, Padh BK. Thalassemia prevention: Religious and cultural barriers to premarital screening in Bangladesh Health Sci Rep. 2023;6(4):e1176.
20. Baxi A, Manila K. Carrier Screening for β Thalassemia in Pregnant Indian Women: Experience at a Single Center in Madhya Pradesh Indian J Hematol Blood Transfus. 2012;29(2):71-4.
21. Kumari S, Seth P. Antenatal screening for thalassemia carrier at tertiary care centre. Home Arch. 2023;12(8).
22. Thaker P, Colah RB, Patel J. Newborn Screening for Sickle Cell Disease Among Tribal Populations in the States of Gujarat and Madhya Pradesh in India: Evaluation and Outcome Over 6 Years. Front Med (Lausanne). 2022;8:731884.
23. Quarmyne MA, Bock F. MPH Newborn Screening for Sickle Cell Disease and Thalassemia. JAMA Health Forum. 2025;6(3):e250064.
24. Balgir RS. The spectrum of hemoglobin variants in two scheduled tribes of Sundargarh district in North-Western Orissa, India. Ann Hum Biol. 2005;32:560-73.
25. Patel AP, Naik MR, Shah NM, et al. Prevalence of common hemoglobinopathies in Gujarat: analysis of a large population screening program. Nat J Community Med. 2012;3:112-6.
26. Chatterjee T, Chakravarti A, Chakravarty S. Population screening and prevention strategies for thalassemias and other hemoglobinopathies of eastern India: experience of 18166 cases. Hemoglobin. 2015;39:384-8.
27. Dolai TK, Dutta S, Bhattacharyya M, et al. Prevalence of hemoglobinopathiein rural Bengal, India. Hemoglobin. 2012;36:57-63.
28. Sonkawade N, Kinikar AA, Kulkarn RK. Screening of Extended Family Members of Thalassemia Major Children as a Thalassemia Preventive Strategy Ethiop J Health Sci. 2022;32(6):1203-10.
29. Agrawal M. Awareness about thalassemia and feasibility of cascade screening in families of thalassemia major patients Home Arch. 2019;6(6).
30. Ministry of Health and Family Welfare, Government of India. Guidelines for National Programme for Prevention and Management of Sickle Cell Disease: National Sickle Cell Anaemia Elimination Mission 2023. New Delhi: Ministry of Health and Family Welfare; 2023.

5

CHAPTER

Community Level Screening/Confirmation; Relevant for National Program

Rabindra Kumar Jena, Sudha Sethy, Amiya Kumar Sahoo

INTRODUCTION

Screening/diagnosis of thalassemia and other hemoglobinopathies at community level is the most challenging one and a need for a different approach in comparison to institutional level. The methodology should be technically correct, practical and sustainable etc. No single strategy can meet the needs of every population. Selection of target population and timing of screening are important determinants for prevention and control strategies as they determine the technical options available for prevention and control, guide community education and counseling needs. Every state can choose the methodology at community level depending on the need and prevailing situation. Screening for early detection of beta-thalassemia (TDT and NTDT) to achieve reduction in mortality and morbidity with improvement in the quality of life of the affected, whereas screening for detection of carrier beta-thalassemia traits to reduce the birth of children affected with thalassemia.

Universal screening for thalassemia major/minor should be done for children (6 months to 6 years). Mass anemia screening will be helpful in identification of thalassemia. Hemoglobin estimation with complete CBC if available/workable could facilitate early diagnosis of thalassemia.

Community screening (Micro Community) by ASHA workers, CHOs and other field workers for severe anemia along with DBS sample collection for HPLC can be the main strategy for early identification/confirmation. Further thalassemia screening/confirmation at facility level can be done through microchip electrophoresis method. However, any alternative viable confirmatory and workable methodology/technology including HPLC/CZE/could be an option depending on the situation.

Population screening for carriers at community level is the mainstay of prevention programs. The greatest challenge in large scale screening is nonavailability of tests with high sensitivity, sustainability, cost effectiveness and implementability at community level. There is no availability of a single screening test which can capture the common hemoglobinopathies prevalent in India i.e., beta thalassemia, HbS and HbE etc. Red cell indices like MCV, RDW, MCH, though sensitive in capturing beta thalassemia trait in institutional laboratories, have missed at community level in 30% of cases due to various reasons. In addition, these parameters are also not available at village and sub center levels due to non-availability of cell counter and lab technicians.

Other screening tests like NESTROFT (Naked Eye SingleTube Red Cell Osmotic Fragility Test), DCIP (Di-Chlorophenol-Indophenol Test, Sickle Solubility Test (Tube Method) meant for beta thalassemia, HbE and HbS respectively are not recommended at present in community level due to high false positive/negative results and cumbersome process. However, point of care test for SCD like HemoType SC/Sickle SCAN/ Indian POCTs based on lateral flow immunoassay are effective with high sensitivity and specificity, albeit only screening for sickle cell disease and missing other types of hemoglobinopathies.

NEWER TECHNOLOGY[1-6]

Microchip Electrophoresis

This technology offers next generation integrated cost-effective and rapid point-of-care solution for detecting beta-thalassemia, sickle cell and HbE in single multiplex test. Using a finger-prick or heel-prick blood sample, it separates hemoglobin variants based on charge differences. The process involves applying the blood sample to a cellulose acetate paper strip, which is then placed in a cartridge and run through a reader. The reader separates, images, and monitors the hemoglobin variants in real time. The test showed 100% sensitivity and specificity in distinguishing beta-thalassemia major/ intermedia from both healthy individuals and those with beta-thalassemia trait. It also demonstrated 100% sensitivity and 98.3% specificity in identifying beta-thalassemia trait compared to healthy subjects in Indian settings.[1] The system is affordable, compact, and portable, enabling decentralized testing and rapid point-of-care results in less than 10 minutes, and can be performed by minimally trained personnel. This technology is being widely used in facilities level of PHC and CHC across Odisha state.

A field study in Tamil Nadu demonstrated that the POCT is valid for identifying thalassemia trait, with a sensitivity of 92.59% and a PPV of 84.74%. This technology can be used for community level one step screening plus confirmatory tests. This technology is empowered with AI enabled automatic results interpretation which minimize the dependency on expert person/hematologist at community level. All consumables can be stored at room temperature and it doesn't need any ancillary instrument for its operation. Several research papers published reveal that this technology might be used for screening and confirmatory tests of thalassemia, SCD and HbE (both trait and homozygous).

Microchip base electrophoresis is fully automated, battery operated, GPS enabled and can be connected with cloud data/server for automatic uploading of the results. This might help to minimize manual error and create a clean database for the test performed.

The same platform can be used to do quantitative Ferritin test (FIA test) by using whole blood samples. This facilitates an integrated approach for further treatment management of thalassemia patients.

DBS-HPLC System[7-11]

The use of dried blood spot (DBS) samples for HPLC analysis (DBS-HPLC) offer a practical yet technically advanced and accurate one-step screening and diagnostic tool for all clinically relevant hemoglobinopathies in large-scale population studies, especially in resource-poor remote locations.

Conventional HPLC systems which require whole blood samples by phlebotomy, transport and storage of samples with challenging logistics and environment. On the contrary, DBS-HPLC requires blood collected through capillary puncture from finger, heel or toe prick. Blood is blotted onto special filter paper, air dried for 1–2 hours and shipped to the lab at ambient temperature for testing. DBS collection requires minimal training, quick and easy to collect via a finger prick and only a few drops of blood are enough for analysis. DBS samples also have an advantage of being robust, remaining suitable for analysis for weeks at ambient temperatures, eliminating the need for special transport and logistics.

DBS samples for hemoglobinopathy screening can be collected by existing healthcare workers with proper training and can be integrated with other national screening programs utilizing finger prick capillary blood, like Anemia Control Program Malaria Control program etc., optimizing use of government resources.

DBS-HPLC accurately identifies and quantifies HbF, HbA, HbA2, HbS, HbE and other Hb-variants in a single 4 minutes run with very high reproducibility for all age groups.

DBS-HPLC is highly sensitive and specific, requires minimal blood, is easy to operate, highly automated with high throughput, and is cost effective on a large scale. This makes DBS-HPLC an ideal technology for population screening.

Use of DBS for HPLC for screening and diagnosis of hemoglobinopathies for all age groups, i.e., Newborns to adults have been validated in studies worldwide. Recently ICMR has validated use of DBS for sickle cell and thalassemia for newborns, children and adults showing 99.3% sensitivity and specificity as compared to whole blood HPLC analysis for sickle cell, thalassemia and other variant hemoglobinopathies.[11] NHM has recently approved the use of DBS sample for HPLC and capillary electrophoresis for all age groups wide in letter dated 3rd June 2024.

Utilizing DBS samples with HPLC provides a one-step screening cum diagnostic test, not just for SCA but for all clinically relevant hemoglobinopathies especially in field setting involving door to door sample collection more so in remote and tribal regions.

DBS-HPLC has been successfully used in Bastar, Chhattisgarh one of the remotest regions of India and in currently being used in seven districts of Odisha for population screening covering of all clinically relevant hemoglobinopathies, i.e., sickle cell, thalassemia, HbE, HbD, other variant hemoglobinopathies and compound heterozygous cases.

Comprehensive Model of Screening/ Confirmation of Thalassemia and Other Hemoglobinopathies

Beta-thalassemia, HbS and HbE are the major hemoglobinopathies (Hb-pathies) seen in India. It is logical to adopt a method which will capture and confirm all common types of Hb-pathies in one-go for optimal utilization of the resources.

- *Technology used*: **Table 1** summarizes the suggested tests at each healthcare level. **Flowchart 1** shows the stepwise approach for confirmation of thalassemia.
    - *Facility-based community level screening and confirmation*: Facility-based community level screening at institution levels such as PHC, UPHC, CHC, UCHC and SDH to screen and confirm by microchip cartridge-based electrophoresis analyzer (Gazelle Device).
    - *Micro-community based universal /opportunistic screening and confirmation*: At micro-community level DBS-HPLC technology is being used for door to door, school level, at anganwadi center, at PMSMA camps, VHND sessions and also at difficult/ hard to reach areas.
    - *Point of care PCR/other newer technology*: States may consider these options depending on their needs and other factors. However, none of such ideal tests are available to be recommended at present.
- *Adoption of implementation partner (PPP model/existing system)*: Total implementation of the program at community level includes training of the healthcare personnel, counseling, patient's registration, sample collection/ transportation/storage/investigation, interpretation of the results and entry of the data in the government portal. This process has a lot of challenges and barriers in the existing healthcare system

TABLE 1: Suggested screening of POCT/confirmation for each level of healthcare.

Healthcare level	POCT/Confirmation suggested	Infrastructural requirement
AAM-SHC-door to door/universal screening/opportunity screening/ fixed day screening/hard to reach areas (community level)	DBS by HPLC/any other suitable method	Central lab with HPLC/any other suitable equipment
Facilities based community level		
AAM-PHC	Microchip electrophoresis	Lab technician with minimal basic skills
CHC	Microchip electrophoresis	Lab technician with minimal basic skills
SDH	Microchip electrophoresis	Lab technician with minimal basic skills
DH	CZE/HPLC	CZE/HPLC lab technician
Medical College	CZE/HPLC, molecular test	Lab with HPLC, CZE and molecular lab

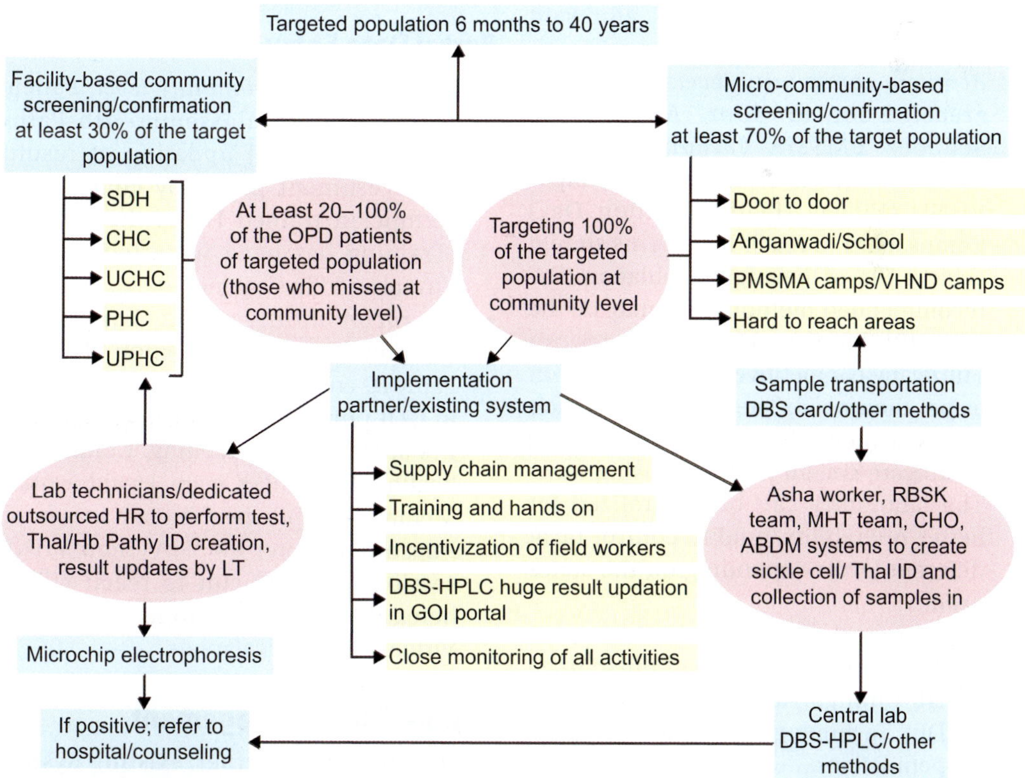

FLOWCHART 1: Confirmation testing strategy for thalassemia and hemoglobinopathies, highlighting the role of HPLC, CZE, microchip electrophoresis, and molecular mutation testing.

across the country. Each state may adopt PPP mode or existing system for optimal implementation of the program. Government of Odisha has adopted PPP mode for implementation.

Methodology at community level: This programme of screening/confirmation can be done by two ways:

1. *At facilities-based community level*: It includes areas of SDH, CHC, UCHC, PHC, UPHC. It may cover 30% of the target population. The recommended methodology is Microchip Electrophoresis (Gazelle) as depicted in the workflow diagram. However, other newer technologies if found suitable to diagnose beta thalassemia and other Hb Pathies can be considered by the state depending on various factors. Government of Odisha has adopted Microchip based Electrophoresis (Gazelle) at aforesaid facilities across the state.
2. *At micro-community level*: It includes areas; Door to door, Anganwadi/ Schools, PMSMA (Pradhan Mantri Surakhita Matrutwa Abhiyan) Camps/ VHND (Village Heath Nutrition Day) Camps, hard to reach areas. This should achieve 70% of the target population. The recommended methodology may be the DBS-HPLC System. However, states can utilize any competitive alternative option as per their need. The sample collection can be achieved by utilizing the existing healthcare system in the following ways. The laboratory can be centralized for better operability/quality control or at different levels depending on the states need.
   - *Door-to-door universal screening* by ASHA worker/dedicated outsourced HR through sample collection with DBS Technology to test 0–40 years of populations.
   - *Collection of DBS samples through Mobile Health Team (RBSK Team)* is being done at school level and Anganwadi centers.
   - *Fixed day testing*: (i) During PMSMA (Pradhan Mantri Surakhita Matrutwa Abhiyan) Platform for antenatal cases once in a month (9th of each month); (ii) during VHND (Village Health Nutritional Day) session DBS sample of antenatal, postnatal and adolescent cases (if missed during door-to-door campaign) by community health officer and Asha worker twice in a week (Tuesday and Friday).
   - *Hard/difficult to reach areas*: DBS samples are an easy and suitable method and should be collected by the mobile health team.
   - States may adopt alternative suitable methodology as deemed fit after considering all the factors.

Portal Data Entry

- *Facility-based community level*: Patient registration (thalassemia-/Hb-Pathy ID creation) and updating of results in government portal by concern lab technician/trained HR of the facilities (Training has been imparted through Virtual and Physical mode)
- *Microcommunity level*: For Micro-Community level registration (Thal/Hb Pathy ID creation) and updating of results in GOI portal by ASHA workers/trained LTs at Universal screening. Community health officer, RBSK team, Health worker (Female), mobile health team at school, Anganwadi center, PMSMA Camp, VHND session hard/difficult to reach village being done through proper training by Virtual and physical mode.

Supply Chain Management

Implementing a partner/existing system supplies the DBS kits to the District HQ. The district in term supplies the same to CHC HQ.

Health worker (Female) concern, collects the same from the CHC HQ on monthly meeting days. The health worker (Female) distributes the same to selected literate AHAS's who were having android mobile phone for Thal/Hb-Pathy ID creation through Hb-Pathy portal mobile application.

MHU and MHT also collect the DBS kit from CHC HQ and utilize the same for the eligible population. Same distribution Channel is being used to return the DBS sample collected to distribution point (CHC HQ), thereon the implementing partner/ existing system collect the DBS sample from the CHC HQ and transport the same to central HPLC lab. The DBS HPLC result of the test entered into the GOI Sickle Cell Portal by the implementing partner/existing system.

Incentives

The fieldworker is being incentivized for portal entry and ID creation @ Rupees five. For transportation of the kit from field to collection point (CHC, SDH, DHS) @Rupees Ten is being given to the AVDM/Non-Android user ASHA's/Health Worker/Community Health Officer. However, the states can modify incentivization as deemed fit.

Confirmation testing: It is preferable to confirm by two alternative confirmatory tests like HPLC/CZE/microchip electrophoresis/ molecular mutation testing/any other suitable test whenever required.

- Mutation testing may be needed to confirm the diagnosis if the patient is transfused and both parents are unavailable or if a difficult case for diagnosis. Mutation testing may be required if prenatal testing is being offered.

CONCLUSION

Community-level screening and diagnosis of thalassemia and hemoglobinopathies require a tiered, context-specific approach for effective implementation. Facility-based microchip electrophoresis (e.g., Gazelle device) and micro-community-based DBS-HPLC systems have proven practical, scalable, and effective in the Indian setting. Integration with existing national screening programs and digital data management portals ensures sustainability, while adoption of PPP models can aid in overcoming infrastructure gaps. Confirmatory testing with at least two standardized modalities, including molecular testing when indicated, ensures diagnostic accuracy. Together, these strategies pave the way for large-scale thalassemia control and effective prevention programs across diverse community settings.

SUMMARY

- Community-level screening for thalassemia and hemoglobinopathies requires context-specific, technically accurate, practical, and sustainable strategies tailored to local conditions.
- Universal screening for thalassemia major/minor should target children aged 6 months to 6 years, integrating anemia screening and early diagnosis.
- Facility-based screening leverages microchip electrophoresis (Gazelle device) for rapid, point-of-care detection of β-thalassemia, HbS, and HbE with high sensitivity and specificity.
- Micro-community-level screening employs DBS-HPLC technology, enabling door-to-door, school, anganwadi, and camp-based outreach, particularly in hard-to-reach areas.
- Microchip electrophoresis offers portability, automation, cloud data connectivity, and AI-enabled interpretation, reducing dependency on specialist personnel.

- DBS-HPLC allows robust, ambient-temperature sample storage and transportation, integrating seamlessly with other national health programs, and achieves high diagnostic accuracy for multiple hemoglobinopathies.
- Confirmatory diagnosis should use at least two modalities, with molecular testing reserved for complex cases, transfused patients, or prenatal diagnostic contexts.
- Effective program implementation depends on trained personnel, incentivized field workers, streamlined supply chain management, portal-based patient registration, and the PPP model for bridging infrastructure gaps.

REFERENCES

1. Piplani S, Kaur M, Madan M. Is NESTROF T better than the hematological indices for screening of beta-thalassemia trait: an answer in rural scenario. Indian J Pathol Oncol. 2017;4:63-70.
2. Ran AN, Avanaki A, Thota P, et al. Point-of-Care Diagnostic Test for Beta-Thalassemia. Biosensors. 2024;14(2):83.
3. Jain A, Jena RK, Dolai TK, et al. Exploring Advances in Point-of-Care Diagnosis: Microchip Electrophoresis for Hemoglobinopathy Detection in Indian Populations. Blood. 2024;144(Supplement 1):3621.
4. Singh N, Seth T, Dass J. Assessment of diagnostic accuracy of Gazelle: A point-of-care testing device for screening β-thalassemia trait. Indian J Med Res. 2024;160:194-200.
5. Canatan D, Delibas S, Altunsoy E, et al. Premarital Screening of Thalassemia and Hemoglobinopathies with Microchip Electrophoresis (Gazelle) Method in a Turkish Population. London: ASCAT 19th Annual Sickle Cell & Thalassaemia Conference; 2024.
6. Shrestha P, Lohse H, Bhatla C, et al. Low-Cost Automated Microscopy and Morphology-Based Machine Learning Classiffication of Sickle Cell Diseaseand Beta-Thalassemia in Nepal and Canada. Blood. 2023;142:790-1.
7. Jena RK, Shetty S, Dash PK, et al. Hemoglobin variant analysis and its comparison between conventional high-performance liquid chromatography using whole blood versus dried blood spot: High-performance liquid chromatography. Indian J Public Health. 2025;69(3);280-5.
8. Roa PD, Turner EA, Aguinaga Mdel P. Hemoglobin variant detection from dried blood specimens by high performance liquid chromatography. Ann Clin Lab Sci. 1993;23(6):433-8.
9. Schaefer BA, Kiyaga C, Howard TA, et al. Hemoglobin variants identified in the Uganda Sickle Surveillance Study. Blood Adv. 2016;1(1): 93-100.
10. Pornprasert S, Kasemrad C, Sukunthamala K. Diagnosis of thalassemia on dried blood spot samples by high performance liquid chromatography. Hemoglobin. 2010;34(5):486-94.
11. ICMR. (2023). File No. 56/02/2023-SCD-TH/ BMS . [online] Available from https://www.icmr.gov.in/icmrobject/custom_data/1720339314_scd_poct_validation_icmr.pdf [Last accessed October,2025].

6

CHAPTER

Molecular Diagnosis of Thalassemia

Reena Das, Prashant Sharma

INTRODUCTION

The diagnosis of thalassemia has traditionally relied on a combination of clinical findings, complete blood count, peripheral smear, and hemoglobin studies using high performance liquid chromatography (HPLC) or capillary electrophoresis (CE), which are sufficient in most symptomatic and carrier states. However, molecular diagnosis has become increasingly important for resolving diagnostic dilemmas, confirming ambiguous laboratory results, and guiding prenatal screening and genetic counseling. Molecular testing not only enables precise mutation detection in both α- and β-thalassemia but also helps in genotype–phenotype correlation, prognostication, and the selection of appropriate therapeutic and preventive strategies. With advances in PCR-based methods, sequencing approaches, and next-generation technologies, molecular testing is now a cornerstone for accurate diagnosis, effective family counseling, and the implementation of preventive programs.

MOLECULAR GENETIC TESTING IN THALASSEMIA

A combination of clinical findings, CBC, blood film examination and hemoglobin studies including high performance liquid chromatography or capillary electrophoresis (HPLC/CE) and, if required, special tests like staining for HbH/fetal hemoglobin, heat/isopropanol stability tests are usually sufficient for the basic diagnosis of all symptomatic forms of thalassemia, i.e., β-thalassemia major (transfusion-dependent β-thalassemia, TDT), β-thalassemia intermedia (nontransfusion-dependent β-thalassemia, NTDT), hemoglobin Bart's hydrops fetalis (α-thalassemia major), and HbH disease (α-thalassemia intermedia).[1,2]

- Similarly, the heterozygous carrier states of genetic importance can also, in the majority of the cases, be identified with certainty using HPLC/CZE, in conjunction with the automated blood counts.[3,4]
- Molecular genetic testing in routine patient care (i.e., outside of a research setting) is indicated in and triggered by either specific clinical situations or in the face of laboratory findings that are ambiguous or require further exploration. These are enumerated in **Box 1** below.

GENERAL PRACTICE POINTS IN GENOTYPIC TESTING IN THALASSEMIC PATIENTS

- Testing of genomic DNA extracted from peripheral blood mononuclear cells of the patient is sufficient for the diagnosis of hemoglobin disorders. DNA from buccal epithelial cells obtained by swabs is also acceptable in very recently transfused patients.[1,10,11]

BOX 1 Indications for molecular genetic testing in thalassemia.[2,5-10]

Clinical indications: Diagnostic dilemma, clinical vs. lab results do not correlate

- In recently transfused patients, where HPLC/CZE do not reveal a clear picture
- For clinically ambiguous cases, or with clinical vs. lab phenotype mismatch. For example:
  - Cases of β-thalassemia intermedia/NTDT
  - β-thalassemia trait with disproportionately severe clinical symptoms
  - Patients in whom parental HPLC/CE testing is not available or not feasible
- In couples at risk of having a baby with a significant (i.e., severely symptomatic) hemoglobin disorder. For example, β-thalassemia major/TDT, severe β-thalassemia intermedia (NTDT), sickle cell anemia, double heterozygosity for sickle/β^0 thalassemia, sickle/HbD-Punjab, etc.)
- Infants where both parents are β-thalassemia trait, and a presumptive diagnosis of β-thalassemia major made on HPLC/CE needs to be confirmed by genetic studies

Laboratory indications:

- Unusual/uncommon hemoglobin variants that remain unexplained even after an independent second-line technique
- Ambiguous HPLC/CE findings insufficient to distinguish double heterozygous states (e.g., sickle/β-thalassemia, HbE/β-thalassemia) from homozygous states (sickle cell anemia or SS-state, HbE disease or EE-state)
- Borderline-high HbA2 (typically defined as HbA2% between 3.4–3.9%, both boundary values being included)
- Unexplained "thalassemic indices" (i.e., erythrocytosis, microcytosis, hypochromia, normal red cell distribution width) in persons with normal range HbA2% (to exclude α-thalassemia trait/silent carrier states).
- Unexplained elevation of fetal hemoglobin

- Even in patients who have been recently transfused with packed red cell units, contamination/microchimerism from allogeneic blood donor-derived leukocytes is unlikely to affect the results of conventional PCR-based genotypic studies, if the blood sample is collected after 24 hours of the transfusion. Caution may, however, be advisable if the patient is markedly leukopenic, and/or freshly collected whole blood was transfused.[12-14]
- In clinically typical cases of transfusion-dependent thalassemia, genetic testing to determine the precise *HBB* mutations (primary modifiers) is desirable but not essential to plan and guide treatment, provided that the diagnosis has been confirmed by the index case's HPLC/CE showing predominantly HbF, markedly reduced adult Hb, and HPLC/CE studies confirm heterozygous carrier status of both parents. However, genetic testing is essential if prenatal diagnostic testing is envisaged in the future.[1,2,10,15,16]
- Determining the *HBB* mutations is desirable, if practically feasible, for a more detailed understanding of the likely clinical course of the patient.[1,2,10,15,16]
- NTDT or β-thalassemia intermedia patients typically benefit from confirmatory molecular testing, with the DNA analysis clarifying the clinical picture, and guiding genetic counseling. Such testing should begin with determination of the *HBB* mutation(s), followed by PCRs or multiplexed-ligation-dependent probe amplification (MLPA) for α-globin gene deletions and/or triplications.[6,7,17-19]
- Symptomatic individuals in whom only a single β-globin gene mutation is detected may have inherited:[6,7,18]
  - Supernumerary α-globin genes
  - Mutations in *HBB* exon 3 (dominant β-thalassemia)

- ○ An unstable hemoglobin
- ○ Another contributing cause for the anemia (e.g., severe forms of G6PD deficiency, hereditary spherocytosis), or a phenocopy of β-thalassemia major/TDT as an altogether different cause for their symptoms (e.g., congenital dyserythropoietic anemia) with the β-thalassemia trait being an incidental finding.
- In all the above genetic testing scenarios, availability of parental screening results, as well as availability of parental DNA specimens, if possible, is valuable in elucidating the cause of symptoms in the proband.[8,19]
- Persons with a $\beta^0\beta^0$ genotype with unexpectedly milder symptoms should undergo testing for concomitant α-thalassemia.[20,21]
- If an NTDT case is still unexplained, testing for polymorphisms influencing HbF levels, like the Xmn1$^{G}\gamma$ -158(C>T) should be done. It often shows linkage of the T genotype to the common IVS 1-1 (G > T) mutation, and may be useful to predict response to HbF-inducing agents.[11,22]
- While genetic testing is not essential to diagnose HbH disease, it can help guide management decisions by distinguishing deletional (mild) forms from non-deletional (typically moderate-to-severe) forms.[23-26]
- Initial testing in HbH disease should include targeted deletion analysis for common *HBA1* and *HBA2* deletions (done by multiplex gap-PCR or MLPA), followed by sequence analysis of the α-globin genes. If the above are normal, the regulatory region multispecies conserved sequence 2 (MCS-R2; previously called HS-40) should be screened for uncommon deletions.[23-26]
- If still unresolved, Sanger sequencing of *HBA2* and *HBA1* genes should be considered.[23-26]

METHODOLOGICAL CONSIDERATIONS IN GENETIC TESTING FOR β-THALASSEMIA[6,9-11,18,19,25,27,28]

- PCR-based amplification refractory mutation system (ARMS) is used in many laboratories because of the simplicity of the assay.
- In ARMS-PCR, a mismatch at the 3′ end of one of the primers prevents the elongation of the primer by Taq polymerase.
- The common primers amplify a 861-bp product that serves as the internal control and also directly detects the presence of the 619 bp deletion (242 bp size), commonly found in Gujarati Indians. Another set of primers which can detect the site of the mutation is added individually in each PCR reaction. A specific product of the desired size shows the presence of the mutation and/or the wild-type allele.
- An alternative method is the reverse dot-blot method where all the three exons are amplified together and blotted on to membranes with the normal and mutant probes spotted as dots. After hybridization of the patient's DNA followed by color development, the spots of the mutants and normal are visualized to interpret the results.
- Sequence analysis of *HBB* using direct DNA sequencing by Sanger method can detect missense, nonsense, and splice site variants and small intragenic insertions/deletions in one test. Despite its high capital costs and technical complexity, its "single test" advantage means that it can be a suitable first-line genetic test in many

situations where individual end-point PCRs are tedious and time-consuming.

- Direct DNA sequencing (Sanger sequencing) will not detect large deletions/duplications involving a single exon, multiple exons, or the whole gene.
- If only one variant or no variant is detected by Sanger sequencing, gene-targeted deletion/duplication analysis should be performed. This is most conveniently done through MLPA.
- *HBD* sequencing is rendered difficult by the presence of its highly homologous gene family members as well as a pseudogene, *HBBP1*.
- Targeted gene panel sequencing, whole exome sequencing or whole genome sequencing by NGS technologies are not considered first-line tests for genetic diagnosis of thalassemia technique due to the small size of the genes being tested, and the high cost of NGS. However, constant evolution of these technologies means that advances in this field are likely in the near future.

PRENATAL DIAGNOSIS OF β-THALASSEMIA: ROLE OF MOLECULAR GENETIC TESTING[15,16,29-35]

- Genetic counseling for prenatal diagnosis is required to decide regarding what would be best for a particular family. It is dependent on many factors such as ethical, legal, social and financial constraints in the particular population.
- Complete assessment and investigation of the couple, well in advance of the pregnancy, allows for timely molecular diagnosis in an unstressed manner. Identifying the exact nature of the genetic abnormality greatly enhances the ability to offer prenatal diagnosis.
- It is important to explain the risks and complications of the fetal sampling procedure, and to inform the couple that the test may be unsuccessful for technical and laboratory reasons or may require a repeat fetal sample (CVS, amniocentesis or cordocentesis).
- It should be clarified to the couple that only specific conditions are being tested, i.e., thalassemia, and a normal result does not guarantee a normal baby (in the event of some other congenital disorder occurring).
- The probability of a misdiagnosis (1–2%) due to various factors, particularly if linkage analysis is used should be explained.
- The fetal sample of choice is the chorionic villous biopsy (CVS) taken at 10–14 weeks of gestation.
- In the second trimester (between 14 and 20 weeks), amniocentesis-derived fetal amniocytes and other cells are used as the source of DNA.
- The third option of using fetal umbilical cord blood obtained through cordocentesis is least popular; and practiced by very few centers.
- For DNA analysis, methods in clinical use are applied as 'direct methods'; that means the mutations of the couple are known and one tests for them in the fetal sample. ARMS-PCR and/or reverse-dot blot PCR are used for known mutations.
- Preimplantation genetic diagnosis (PGD) approach has been developed for prenatal diagnosis of several genetic disorders including β-thalassemia and hemoglobinopathies. In this, the congenital disorder is avoided through selection of unaffected gametes or embryos before pregnancy. This in vitro process offers the advantage of avoiding an abortion. For PGD, the sample analyzed is a polar body or a single cell taken from 4–8 cell blastomeres. DNA is extracted from the single cell and PCR performed for the mutations in case of β-thalassemia.[36,37]

- Cell-free fetal DNA from maternal plasma is currently being technically refined for obtaining DNA as a noninvasive method. In autosomal recessive disorders like thalassemia, it is more difficult to rule out maternal contamination. However, the absence of the paternal mutation would indicate the fetus is either heterozygous or normal. It is challenging when both the partners have the same mutation.[30,38,39]

MOLECULAR GENETICS AND GENOTYPE-PHENOTYPE CORRELATION IN NTDT/THALASSEMIA INTERMEDIA[6-8,17,18,22,40]

NTDT arises from gene function defects that lead to only partial suppression of β-globin protein production. Most NTDT patients are homozygotes or compound heterozygotes for β-thalassemia where both β-globin loci are affected. Less frequently, only a single β-globin locus is affected.

The milder clinical characteristics of NTDT compared with TDT occur primarily due to three different mechanisms which are:

- *Inheritance of a mild or silent β-chain mutation*: The level of synthesis of β-chains is subnormal rather than being completely absent. This causes a reduced imbalance between the numbers of α- and β-chains thus ameliorating the phenotype (β+/β++).
- *Coinheritance of determinants associated with increased γ-globin chain production*: The increase in the number of γ chains helps to neutralize the large proportion of free α-chains.
- *Coinheritance of α-thalassemia*: This helps to suppress the synthesis of α-chains again leading to reduction of α-/β-chain imbalance.

Common genetic interactions underlying the phenotype of NTDT are enumerated in **Box 2**.

Mild β-thalassemia Mutations

Most β-thalassemia mutations lead to a total absence or severe reduction of β-globin chain

BOX 2 **Genotypes of NTDT classified based on whether one or both the HBB alleles are affected in a patient.**[6-8,17,18,22,40-43]

- *Homozygous or compound heterozygous states for β-thalassemia*:
  - Inheritance of mild β-thalassemia alleles, β "silent" and β++, in homozygous or compound heterozygous states:
    - Coinheritance of α-thalassemia with two β^0 alleles
    - Increased HbF response due to any of the following:
      - ◊ Xmn1Gγ polymorphism
      - ◊ HBB promoter mutations
  - *Transacting* quantitative trait loci (QTLs) for HbF on Xp22.2-p22.3, 6q23, 8q, and 2p15
- *Heterozygous state for β-thalassemia*:
  - Coinheritance of additional α-globin genes (ααα/αα, ααα/ααα, αααα/αα, αααα/αααα): This exacerbates the phenotypic severity of β-thalassemia by causing more globin chain imbalance (Weatherall DJ,1998; Weatherall DJ, 2001).
    - Dominantly inherited β-thalassemia (hyperunstable β-globin chain variants)
    - Somatic deletion of the other β-globin locus—mosaicism
- *Compound heterozygotes* for β-thalassemia and β-globin chain variants, e.g., HbE/ β-thalassemia

synthesis. Mild β-thalassemia mutations have a less severe reduction in the synthesis of normal β-globin chains. Several mutations located at positions upstream of the β-globin gene lead to mild to moderately reduced transcriptional output (β++ type). These include the –88 (C > T) mutations in Asian Indians and American Blacks, –101 (C > T) in Mediterranean groups and Italians, –28 (A > G) in Chinese, –29 (A > G) in the Black population, and the Cap site +1 (A > C) mutation in Asian Indians.[44-46] Mild β+ mutations are also found in the consensus sequence required for polyadenylation.[9,41,47]

GENOTYPE-PHENOTYPE CORRELATION IN α-THALASSEMIA[21,25,26,48]

- Nondeletional α-thalassemia is typically more severe than deletional variants. Deletions of the *HBA2* gene are more severe than those of *HBA1*.
- Hb Bart's hydrops fetalis most often results from large deletions on both chromosomes (--/--), and only rarely from a nondeletion variant (--/α^{ND}-).
- HbH disease usually occurs due to a large α^0 deletion of one allele in *trans* with either a single α-globin-gene deletional (--/-α) or a nondeletion null variant (--/$\alpha^{ND}\alpha$ or --/$\alpha\alpha^{ND}$).
- Rarely, HbH disease occurs due to homozygosity for nondeletional *HBA2* mutations ($\alpha^{ND}\alpha/\alpha^{ND}\alpha$), or due to homozygosity or compound heterozygosity for highly unstable α-globin gene variants. A commonly encountered nondeletional α-thalassemic mutation in India is *HBA2*:c.314G>A, p.Cys>Tyr (Hb Sallanches).
- The tertiary modifiers are largely common across β- and α-thalassemias.

CONCLUSION

Molecular diagnosis of thalassemia has transformed patient care by providing definitive characterization of mutations, resolving ambiguous clinical and hematological findings, and guiding reproductive decision-making. While traditional hematological tests remain effective for first-line diagnosis, molecular tools are essential for precise detection of complex genotypes, confirmation of NTDT or α-thalassemia variants, and prenatal or preimplantation genetic diagnosis. Understanding genotype–phenotype interactions enhances prediction of disease severity and helps tailor individualized management. As sequencing technologies advance and become more cost-effective, molecular testing will increasingly integrate into routine clinical practice, playing a pivotal role in both patient management and prevention strategies for thalassemia worldwide.

SUMMARY

1. *Primary diagnosis*: Most symptomatic and carrier forms of thalassemia can be diagnosed using clinical assessment, CBC, blood film, HPLC/CE, and select special tests (e.g., HbH stain, instability tests) without molecular testing.
2. *Indications for genetic testing*: Molecular testing is reserved for complex clinical situations (e.g., ambiguous phenotypes, recent transfusions, lack of parental data) or inconclusive lab findings (e.g., borderline HbA2, unexplained HbF elevation, undetected variants).
3. *Specimen for DNA testing*: Peripheral blood is preferred; buccal swabs are acceptable, even post-transfusion. Leukocyte contamination from transfusion is rarely significant if sampled after 24 hours.

4. *NTDT evaluation*: Genetic testing is especially useful in NTDT (non-transfusion-dependent β-thalassemia) to confirm diagnosis, clarify genotype-phenotype correlations, and guide counseling.
5. *NTDT mechanisms*: NTDT results from mild β-mutations, increased γ-globin synthesis (e.g., via Xmn1 polymorphism), and/or coinherited α-thalassemia—modulating α/β chain imbalance and phenotype severity.
6. *Symptomatic heterozygotes*: Individuals with only one detectable β-globin mutation may have additional factors—extra α-globin genes, unstable hemoglobins, dominant mutations, or coexisting disorders (e.g., G6PD deficiency, CDA).
7. *α-Thalassemia genetics*: HbH disease and Hb Bart's hydrops fetalis result from varying combinations of α-globin deletions and mutations; genetic testing distinguishes mild (deletional) from severe (nondeletional) forms.
8. *Methods overview*: ARMS-PCR, reverse dot blot, and Sanger sequencing are commonly used. MLPA is needed for detecting deletions/duplications. NGS is not first-line but holds future potential.
9. *Prenatal diagnosis*: Requires early genetic counseling and preconception carrier identification. Options include CVS (10–14 weeks), amniocentesis (14–20 weeks), cordocentesis, and PGD; cfDNA is under development but technically challenging.
10. *Genotype-phenotype correlation*: Non-deletional α-thalassemia mutations are generally more severe than deletional ones. Molecular testing refines prediction of clinical severity in both α- and β-thalassemias.

REFERENCES

1. Munkongdee T, Chen P, Winichagoon P, et al. Update in Laboratory Diagnosis of Thalassemia. Front Mol Biosci. 2020;7:74.
2. Farmakis D, Porter J, Taher A, et al. 2021 Thalassaemia International Federation Guidelines for the Management of Transfusion-dependent Thalassemia. Hemasphere. 2022;6(8):e732.
3. Mohanty D, Colah RB, Gorakshakar AC, et al. Prevalence of β-thalassemia and other haemoglobinopathies in six cities in India: a multicentre study. J Community Genet. 2013;4(1):33-42.
4. Sharma P, Das R. Cation-exchange high-performance liquid chromatography for variant hemoglobins and HbF/A2: What must hematopathologists know about methodology? World J Methodol. 2016;6(1):20-4.
5. Viprakasit V, Ekwattanakit S. Clinical Classification, Screening and Diagnosis for Thalassemia. Hematol Oncol Clin North Am. 2018;32(2):193-211.
6. Galanello R, Origa R. Beta-thalassemia. Orphanet J Rare Dis. 2010;5:11.
7. Sundaresan DD, Hira JK, Chhabra S, et al. Hematological and genetic profiles of persons with co-inherited heterozygous β-thalassemia and supernumerary α-globin genes. Eur J Haematol. 2023;110(5):510-7.
8. Singh N, Hira JK, Chhabra S, et al. β-thalassemia intermedia mimicking β-thalassemia trait: The importance of family studies and HBB genotyping in phenotypically ambiguous cases. Int J Lab Hematol. 2023;45(4):609-12.
9. Rangan A, Sharma P, Dadu T, et al. β-Thalassemia mutations in subjects with borderline HbA_2 values: a pilot study in North India. Clin Chem Lab Med. 2011;49(12):2069-72.
10. Sabath DE. The role of molecular diagnostic testing for hemoglobinopathies and thalassemias. Int J Lab Hematol. 2023;45(Suppl 2):71-8.
11. Tesio N, Bauer D. Molecular Basis and Genetic Modifiers of Thalassemia. Hematol Oncol Clin North Am. 2023;37(2):273-99.
12. Gong MN, Sai Y, Zhou W, et al. Genotyping Patients with Recent Blood Transfusions. Epidemiology. 2003;14(6):744-7.
13. DiGuardo MA, Kester SJ, Mahaffey VJ, et al. Does Transfusion of Red Blood Cells Impact Germline Genetic Test Results? J Pers Med. 2020;10(4):268.
14. Lee TH, Paglieroni T, Ohto H, et al. Survival of donor leukocyte subpopulations in immunocompetent

transfusion recipients: frequent long-term microchimerism in severe trauma patients. Blood. 1999;93(9):3127-39.
15. Mensah C, Sheth S. Optimal strategies for carrier screening and prenatal diagnosis of α- and β-thalassemia. Hematology Am Soc Hematol Educ Program. 2021;2021(1):607-13.
16. Li DZ, Yang YD. Invasive prenatal diagnosis of fetal thalassemia. Best Pract Res Clin Obstet Gynaecol. 2017;39:41-52.
17. Vichinsky E. Non-transfusion-dependent thalassemia and thalassemia intermedia: epidemiology, complications, and management. Curr Med Res Opin. 2016;32(1):191-204.
18. Galanello R. Recent advances in the molecular understanding of non-transfusion-dependent thalassemia. Blood Rev. 2012;26(Suppl 1:)S7-11.
19. Sharma N, Das R, Kaur J, et al. Evaluation of the genetic basis of phenotypic heterogeneity in north Indian patients with thalassemia major. Eur J Haematol. 2010;84(6):531-7.
20. Saha D, Chowdhury PK, Panja A, et al. Effect of deletions in the α-globin gene on the phenotype severity of β-thalassemia. Hemoglobin. 2022;46(2):118-23.
21. Sripichai O, Munkongdee T, Kumkhaek C, et al. Coinheritance of the different copy numbers of alpha-globin gene modifies severity of beta-thalassemia/Hb E disease. Ann Hematol. 2008;87(5):375-9.
22. Oberoi S, Das R, Panigrahi I, et al. Xmn1-G g polymorphism and clinical predictors of severity of disease in β-thalassemia intermedia. Pediatr Blood Cancer. 2011;57(6):1025-8.
23. Mallik N, Singh N, Jamwal M, et al. A novel ATRX splice variant causing acquired HbH disease in myelodysplastic syndrome with excess blasts-1. Cancer Genet. 2022;260-261:53-6.
24. Sharma P, Das R, Khadwal AR, et al. HbH disease due to compound heterozygosity for hemoglobins Zürich-Albisrieden and Sallanches. Pediatr Blood Cancer. 2020;67(4):e28161.
25. Motiani A, Zubair M, Sonagra AD. Laboratory Evaluation of Alpha Thalassemia. In: StatPearls [Internet]. Treasure Island (FL): StatPearls Publishing; 2025.
26. Tan AS, Quah TC, Low PS, et al. A rapid and reliable 7-deletion multiplex polymerase chain reaction assay for alpha-thalassemia. Blood. 2001;98(1):250-1.
27. Clark BE, Shooter C, Smith F, et al. Next-generation sequencing as a tool for breakpoint analysis in rearrangements of the globin gene clusters. Int J Lab Hematol. 2017;39(Suppl 1):111-20.
28. Zulkeflee RH, Bahar R, Abdullah M, et al. Application of Targeted Next-generation Sequencing for the Investigation of Thalassemia in a Developing Country: A Single Center Experience. Diagnostics (Basel). 2023;13(8):1379.
29. Bandyopadhyay A, Bandyopadhyay S, Basak J, et al. Profile of beta-thalassemia in eastern India and its prenatal diagnosis. Prenat Diagn. 2004;24(12):992-6.
30. Colah RB, Gorakshakar AC, Nadkarni AH. Invasive & non-invasive approaches for prenatal diagnosis of haemoglobinopathies: experiences from India. Indian J Med Res. 2011;134(4):552-60.
31. Gorakshakar AC, Lulla CP, Nadkarni AH, et al. Prenatal diagnosis of beta-thalassemia among Indians using denaturing gradient gel electrophoresis. Hemoglobin. 1997;21(5):421-35.
32. Kabra M. Prenatal diagnosis. Indian J Pediatr. 2003;70(1):81-5.
33. Kumar R, Panigrahi I, Dalal A, et al. Sickle cell anemia--molecular diagnosis and prenatal counseling: SGPGI experience. Indian J Pediatr. 2012;79(1):68-74.
34. Tamhankar PM, Agarwal S, Arya V, et al. Prevention of homozygous beta thalassemia by premarital screening and prenatal diagnosis in India. Prenat Diagn. 2009;29(1):83-8.
35. Patel AP, Patel RB, Patel SA, et al. β-Thalassemia mutations in Western India: outcome of prenatal diagnosis in a hemoglobinopathies project. Hemoglobin. 2014;38(5):329-34.
36. Ren Z, Huang P, Wang Y, et al. Technically feasible solutions to challenges in preimplantation genetic testing for thalassemia: experiences of multiple centers between 2019 and 2022. J Assist Reprod Genet. 2024;41(11):3225-35.
37. Traeger-Synodinos J. Pre-implantation genetic diagnosis. Best Pract Res Clin Obstet Gynaecol. 2017;39:74-88.
38. Liu D, Nong C, Lai F, et al. Research Progress of Cell-free Fetal DNA in Non-invasive Prenatal Diagnosis of Thalassemia. Hemoglobin. 2023;47(2):80-4.
39. Lo YMD, Chiu RWK. Noninvasive approaches to prenatal diagnosis of hemoglobinopathies using fetal DNA in maternal plasma. Hematol Oncol Clin North Am. 2010;24(6):1179-86.
40. Lai Y, Zhou L, Yi S, et al. The association between four SNPs (rs7482144, rs4671393, rs28384513 and rs4895441) and fetal hemoglobin levels in Chinese Zhuang β-thalassemia intermedia patients. Blood Cells Mol Dis. 2017;63:52-7.
41. Thein SL. The molecular basis of β-thalassemia. Cold Spring Harb Perspect Med. 2013;3(5):a011700.

42. Thein SL. Pathophysiology of beta thalassemia--α guide to molecular therapies. Hematology Am Soc Hematol Educ Program. 2005;31-7.
43. Thein SL. Genetic modifiers of beta-thalassemia. Haematologica. 2005;90(5):649-60.
44. Garewal G, Das R, Awasthi A, et al. The clinical significance of the spectrum of interactions of CAP+1 (A-->C), a silent beta-globin gene mutation, with other beta-thalassemia mutations and globin gene modifiers in north Indians. Eur J Haematol. 2007;79(5):417-21.
45. Garewal G, Das R, Ahluwalia J, et al. Nucleotide -88 (C-T) promoter mutation is a common beta-thalassemia mutation in the Jat Sikhs of Punjab, India. Am J Hematol. 2005;79(4):252-6.
46. Sharma P, Das R, Trehan A, et al. Impact of iron deficiency on hemoglobin A2% in obligate β-thalassemia heterozygotes. Int J Lab Hematol. 2015;37(1):105-11.
47. Belisário AR, Sales RR, Viana MB. Very mild forms of Hb S/beta(+)-thalassemia in Brazilian children. Rev Bras Hematol Hemoter. 2015;37(3):198-201.
48. Wang W, Ma ESK, Chan AYY, et al. Single-tube multiplex-PCR screen for anti-3.7 and anti-4.2 alpha-globin gene triplications. Clin Chem. 2003;49(10):1679-82.

7

CHAPTER

Guideline for Prenatal Diagnosis of Thalassemia

Sila Chakrabarti, Jyoti Shaw

INTRODUCTION

Thalassemia is a common inherited blood disorder in India caused by mutations in the β-globin gene, leading to severe anemia and dependence on lifelong transfusions. Prenatal diagnosis (PND) plays a vital role in preventing the birth of affected children by identifying the thalassemia status of the fetus early in pregnancy. Successful PND requires early detection of carrier status in both parents, proper genetic counseling, and the use of reliable molecular techniques such as ARMS-PCR and DNA sequencing to confirm mutations.

URGENT NEED FOR PRENATAL DIAGNOSIS OF THALASSEMIA

Prenatal diagnosis becomes an important option only when both the biological mother and father are carriers of beta thalassemia.

Who will Require PND?

Prenatal diagnosis has currently come up as an important method for prevention of the birth of a thalassemic child, but to make a success of it, early identification of the carrier status of both parents and proper counseling is extremely important. The carrier status of both partners has varied implications for the genetic makeup and health outcome of their baby **(Fig. 1)**.

GENETIC COUNSELING

- The genetic counselors play a very important role as they have the responsibility to counsel the pregnant mother and her husband.
- The "at risk" couple should be counseled together so that they can both have their queries answered and have no room for confusion later on.
- They must be spoken to in a communicable and simple language so that they know that in each pregnancy there is only a 25% chance of getting an affected child in which case they should opt for MTP and this 25% chance will be present in each pregnancy so they would have to go for PND every time the mother becomes pregnant to determine the risk of thalassemia in the fetus.
- The mother and father must be made aware that there is a small (2%) chance of misdiagnosis due to technical error rate.
- It is imperative that the prospective mother and father give their informed consent after knowing the risk factors including the very small risk of abortion

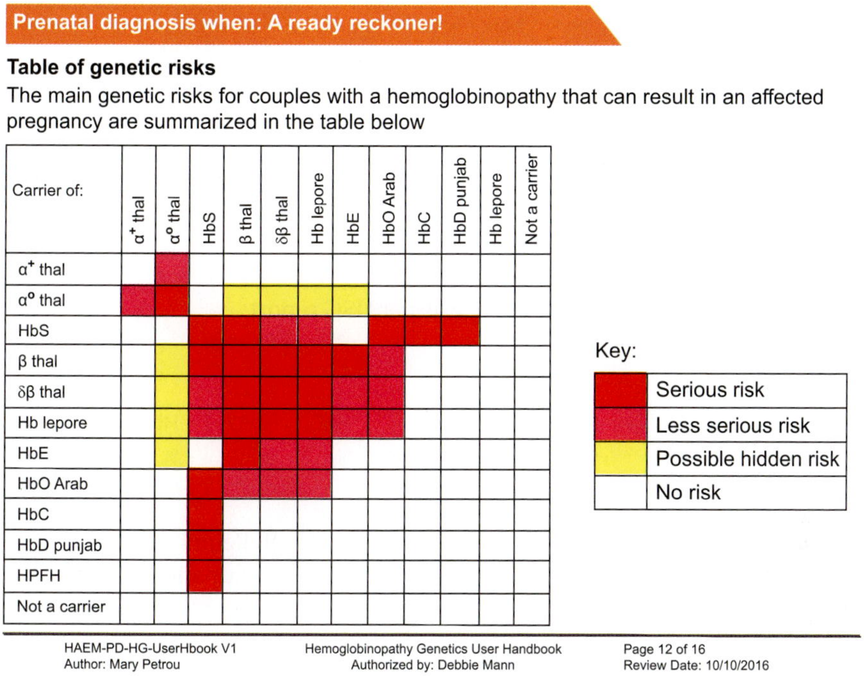

Prenatal diagnosis when: A ready reckoner!

Table of genetic risks

The main genetic risks for couples with a hemoglobinopathy that can result in an affected pregnancy are summarized in the table below

Carrier of:	α+ thal	α° thal	HbS	β thal	δβ thal	Hb lepore	HbE	HbO Arab	HbC	HbD punjab	Hb lepore	Not a carrier
α+ thal		Less serious risk										
α° thal	Less serious risk	Serious risk		Possible hidden risk	Possible hidden risk	Possible hidden risk	Possible hidden risk					
HbS			Serious risk	Serious risk	Less serious risk	Less serious risk		Serious risk	Serious risk	Serious risk		
β thal		Possible hidden risk	Serious risk	Serious risk	Serious risk	Serious risk	Serious risk	Less serious risk				
δβ thal		Possible hidden risk	Less serious risk	Serious risk	Serious risk	Serious risk	Less serious risk	Less serious risk				
Hb lepore		Possible hidden risk	Less serious risk	Serious risk	Serious risk	Serious risk	Less serious risk	Less serious risk				
HbE		Possible hidden risk		Serious risk	Less serious risk	Less serious risk						
HbO Arab			Serious risk	Less serious risk	Less serious risk	Less serious risk						
HbC			Serious risk									
HbD punjab			Serious risk									
HPFH			Serious risk									
Not a carrier												

Key:
- Serious risk
- Less serious risk
- Possible hidden risk
- No risk

HAEM-PD-HG-UserHbook V1 Author: Mary Petrou | Hemoglobinopathy Genetics User Handbook Authorized by: Debbie Mann | Page 12 of 16 Review Date: 10/10/2016

FIG. 1: The main genetic risks for couples with a hemoglobinopathy that can result in an affected pregnancy.

after obtaining CVS/amniotic fluid sample.

The mother and father should both sign a consent form before the samples are sent for DNA analysis.

- Consent forms must be available in Hindi, English as well as the local language for the parents. A general format for the same is given below.

Consent Form

1. We (Names of both husband and wife in block letters as per ID) have been diagnosed as carriers of haemoglobinopathies
2. We have been counseled about the considerable risk of our begetting a child with thalassemia which can be avoided if we opt for antenatal diagnosis by DNA analysis.
3. The entire procedure of CVS sampling/amniotic fluid collection followed by laboratory diagnosis has been explained to us in detail.
4. We are aware of the risks involved of spontaneous abortion following the procedure and the occasional problem of inability to obtain a sample for diagnosis.
5. We are aware that there is a small chance (about 2%) of laboratory misdiagnosis due to unavoidable random error rate present for all kinds of laboratory diagnosis.
6. After considering all these factors we are giving our consent to carry out the prenatal diagnosis of our unborn child.

Signature of Mother with date

Name and address

Signature of Father with date.

Name and address

Requisition Form

All information regarding the mother and father must be noted in a form so that it is easily accessible by the laboratory and stored in the Achieves. The following information is essential:

a. Mother's name: Age: Religion:
Aadhaar No: Occupation:
Address and contact phone number:
Parity: Family history:
LMP: Gestational age as per USG report:
Transfusion history:
HPLC report:

Hb g/dL	RBC 10^{12}/L	MCV Fl	MCH Pg	RDW CV	Hb A2%	Hb A^0%	HbF %	HbA2+E %	HbS %	HbD %	Other

b. Father's name: Age: Religion:
Aadhaar No: Occupation:
Transfusion history:
HPLC report

Hb g/dL	RBC 10^{12}/L	MCV Fl	MCH Pg	RDW CV	Hb A2%	Hb A^0%	HbF %	HbA2+E %	HbS %	HbD %	Other

TABLE 1: Common seven mutations.

Name	Mutation	Nomenclature
IVS1-5(G-C)	Beta nt 147 G>C	HBB:c.92+5G>C
HbE	26(B8) Glu>Lys	HBB:c.79G>A
HbS	Beta 6(A3)Glu>Val	HBBc.20A.>T
Codon30(G-C)	Beta 30(B12) Arg>Thr	HBB:c.92G>C
F41-42(-CTTT)	Beta 41-42(-TTCT) modified terminal sequence	HBB C 126-129 del CTTT
CD15(G-A)	Beta 15(A12) Trp>Stop	HBB:c.47G>A
FS 8/9(+G)	Beta 9(+)G modified C terminal sequence	HBB c.27-28ins(G).

PARENTAL MUTATION

Parental mutations should be checked preferably before conception.

If pregnant then as soon as pregnancy is confirmed they must be sent to the molecular laboratory for mutation detection.

2–3 mL of EDTA blood is collected from each parent for mutation detection.

Routine molecular diagnostic methods like ARMS PCR and/or Reverse Dot Blot(RDB) are used as the first line of work to identify the parental mutations.

Initially seven common mutations to be screened **(Table 1)**.

If mutation is not detected by these the second panel of mutations may be checked by ARMS PCR as they are present in a much lower frequency **(Table 2)**.

However the mutation profile of carriers vary from one region of country to another. So local data if any should be given preference

IF MUTATION NOT IDENTIFIED BY ARMS PCR—SEQUENCING

In the absence of common mutations not detected by ARMS PCR in any one of the parents the mutation has to be identified by Sanger Sequencing before proceeding for prenatal diagnosis. Routine use of Sanger Sequencing methods for mutation detection for all samples in general is considerably more expensive both in terms of consumables and infrastructure so all samples are usually not subjected to Sanger Sequencing. It is however the method of choice for identifying the rare mutations and in case of any clinical doubt

HBB gene sequencing steps:

1. Target DNA fragment (e.g., 953bp) is amplified by PCR method using specified primers
2. Then the result of the PCR is checked by agarose gel electrophoresis. (size of DNA band, primer dimers, presence of smears).
3. Cleaning of PCR product using exonuclease and alkaline phosphatase (Exo-SAP)
4. Sequencing PCR is done using fluorophore tagged dideoxy NTPs (ddNTPs)

TABLE 2: Extended panel of mutations.

Common name	Mutation	Nomenclature
IVS1-1(G-T)	Beta nt 143 G>T	HBB:c.92+1G>T
619 bp deletion	Beta nts 1065 - 1683 deleted	NG_000007.3:g.71609_72227del619
CD16(-C)	Beta 16 (-C); modified C-terminal sequence: (16)Gly-(17)Arg-COOH	HBB:c.51delC
Cap site +1(A-C)	Beta nt 1 A>C	HBB:c.-50A>C
IVS1-(3'end)-25 bp deletion	Beta nts 252 - 276 deleted	HBB:c.93-22_95del
CD30(G-A)	Beta 30(B12) Arg>Lys	HBB:c.92G>A
IVS1-1(G-A)	Beta nt 143 G>A	HBB:c.92+1G>A
IVSII-837(T-G)	Beta nt 1332 T>G	HBB:c.316-14T>G
CD5(-CT)	Beta 5 (-CT); modified C-terminal sequence: (5)Arg-Gly-Glu-Val-Cys-Arg-Tyr-Cys-Pro-Val- Gly-Gln-Gly-Glu-Arg-(20)Gly-COOH	HBB:c.17_18delCT
IVSII-1(G-A)	Beta nt 496 G>A	HBB:c.315+1G>A
IVSII-745(C-G)	Beta nt 1240 C>G	HBB:c.316-106C>G
-88(C-T)	Beta nt -88 C>T	HBB:c.-138C>T
IVSII-654(G-T)	Beta nt 1149 C>T	HBB:c.316-185C>T
IVS1-6(T-C)	Beta nt 148 T>C	HBB:c.92+6T>C
CD39(C-T)	Beta 39(C5) Gln>Stop	HBB:c.118C>T
δβAsian Indian Inversion Deletion Mutation	Deletion of 32624nts from the Delta gene to the beta gene.	NG_000007.3g5050983170del 113666
HPFH3 Indian	Deletion of 49733 nts from HBBP1 gene to beta gene	NG_000007.3:g.53390_103157d el49768

5. Post cleaning of cycle sequencing products by Ethanol and Sodium acetate method
6. Suspending the PCR product in Hi-Di formamide
7. Loading the sample in a DNA Sequencer machine.

Some rare mutations identified by *HBB* gene sequencing by following the above method in the β-thalassemia cohort are summarized below **(Table 3)**.

Implementation and Accomplishment

To implement *HBB* gene sequencing for prenatal diagnosis of thalassemia, sequencing must be done in nodal centers only and there must be sequencing facilities available in the nodal center in each state. In case of ARMS PCR failure, blood samples are sent to the nodal center immediately since DNA sequencing is a multistep process and time consuming. Cases where mutation is identified by DNA sequencing method, CVS sample to be sent directly for DNA sequencing. Hence, adopting this strategy will achieve a thalassemia free nation in near future.

Sample Collection—CVS/Amniotic Fluid

Once the mutations are confirmed the parents are requested to provide the CVS samples or ascertain the thalassemia status of the fetus at the earliest.

Every district hospital should have a trained gynecologist for collection of CVS sample.

CVS samples are collected into sterile plastic conical tubes containing sterile transport medium labeled with Patient's name and ID number.

A completed test requisition form providing the necessary details like Patient's name, ID number, address parental mutation identification result, etc., must be included with every sample.

TABLE 3: Rare mutations identified by *HBB* gene sequencing.

Mutation Name	HGVS nomenclature	Phenotype class
-86 (C>G)	HBB: c-136C>G	β^+
-90 (C>T)	HBB: c-140C>T	β^+
Beta nt -42(C>G)	HBB: c-92C>G	β^+
Capsite +1(A>C)	HBB: c-50A>C	β^+
Hb Stockholm	HBB: C24G>T	Hb variant
HbD Iran	HBB: C67G>C	Hb variant
HbM Saskatoon	HBB: C190C>T	Hb variant
Hb Randwick	HBB: C46T>G	Hb variant
IVS-1-130 (G>C)	HBB: C93-1G>C	β^0
IVS-11-848 (C>A)	HBB: C316-3C>A	β^+
CD10 (C>A)	HBB: C33C>A	β^+
CD 82 (A>T)	HBB: C247A>T	β^0
rs713040	HBB: C9T>C	SNP
IVS-11-16	HBB: C315=16G>C	SNP
IVS-11-666	HBB: C316-18C>T	SNP

Once collected CVS samples must be sent to the molecular diagnostic lab within 1-2 days.

Advantage of CVS Over Amniotic Fluid

Though obtaining an adequate sample of amniotic fluid has the advantage of being a relatively easier procedure technically and it can be obtained in later gestational period compared to CVS sample still CVS is the preferred sample of choice for most molecular diagnostic labs as it is done earlier in pregnancy at 9-13 weeks and provides an appreciably greater yield of DNA to work with compared to uncultured amniocytes thereby allowing reliable DNA analysis within days of sampling with concomitant advantages and the comparable anticipation of results reduce couple anxiety and allow pregnancy termination at a safer gestational time resulting in better maternal wellbeing. Amniotic fluid samples differ considerably in the yield of fetal cells obtained and sometimes the number of fetal cells obtained from amniotic fluid is so small that it becomes very challenging to get the desired result from downstream procedures like PCR if using uncultured amniocytes and often the amount is inadequate if it becomes necessary to repeat an experiment in case of any doubt by the lab personnel.

PROCESSING OF CVS/AMNIOTIC FLUID SAMPLE

CVS samples are first cleaned carefully under a dissecting microscope to separate it from any contaminating maternal tissue. This is an important step for obtaining error free final results.

DNA is next isolated from the cleaned CVS samples using a good quality DNA isolation kit and the quality and quantity is checked using a nano drop spectrophotometer.

The next step is to check the presence of the parental mutations using PCR ARMS and determine whether the fetus is heterozygous/homozygous/compound heterozygous or free from the parental mutations. The tests are carried out more than once to get the same result on two separate days.

CHECKING FOR THE PRESENCE OF MATERNAL CONTAMINATION

Due to potential presence of maternal blood the fetal specimens like CVS and amniotic fluid are at risk of maternal cell contamination (MCC) which poses a risk of prenatal misdiagnosis. The MCC may result in a false positive diagnosis leading to inappropriate pregnancy management. Therefore to obtain test results of higher accuracy to ensure that prenatal samples are considerably free of MCC analysis is carried out using Variable Number of Tandem Repeats (VNTR) in most PND labs.

The highly polymorphic DNA sequence D1S80 VNTR locus is used to monitor MCC in fetal samples. Sequencing of the flanking regions of the 16 nucleotide repeats located on the short arm of chromosome 1 enabled the design of primers by PCR. There are 16 alleles with a repeat pattern of 16 base pairs with allele length range of 387-723 bp and heterozygosity of 0.76.

However D1S80 alone may not provide sufficient information due to either presence of homozygosity of the VNTR in the maternal tissue so some additional informative VNTR markers are required.

The APO B VNTR locus is located on the transcriptional termination signal of the APO B protein gene on chromosome 2. Its core sequence is 14-16 bp in length and consists of AT rich sequence and the allele members vary from 29-55 with heterozygosis of 0.79.

Some of the other VNTR loci for PND of thalassemia are ACTBP2,Ig-JH, TPO, Ha-ras, etc.

Ideally speaking, the VNTR markers suitable for PND in different population groups in India should be determined and a consensus is to be reached for the less common VNTR markers to be used for monitoring of MCC in PND of thalassemia.

Counseling of parents if the in utero baby is affected.

- Parents should be informed about the consequences of having this child
- Counselor should give the options and guide
- Should not be directive

FOLLOW-UP

The patients are requested to check the carrier status of the child by HPLC from peripheral blood samples at >1 years of age of the child though the common recommendation is to repeat and cross check the results from cord blood collected at birth of the child. This is as many of the patients come from far flung and remote villages and these places are ill equipped to collect the cord blood and the parents families do not have the means to reach the samples to the nodal centers and cord blood will also be predominantly HBF so that mutation analysis is a must even for a preliminary idea. Comparatively, this policy is more feasible and acceptable to the parents.

CONCLUSION

Prenatal diagnosis is a crucial preventive measure to reduce the burden of thalassemia major. Early carrier screening, effective counseling, and standardized molecular testing help at-risk couples make informed reproductive decisions. Strengthening PND programs and ensuring their availability at nodal centers can significantly contribute to achieving the goal of a thalassemia-free nation.

SUMMARY

- Prenatal diagnosis (PND) of thalassemia is essential when both parents are carriers, enabling early detection of the fetus's genetic status and preventing the birth of an affected child.
- Effective PND relies on early parental carrier screening, thorough genetic counseling, and obtaining informed consent using formats available in Hindi, English, and local languages.
- Genetic counselors must explain risks clearly, including the 25% recurrence probability in each pregnancy and the small (~2%) chance of technical misdiagnosis.
- Initial mutation identification uses ARMS-PCR for the seven most common β-globin mutations, followed by an extended panel for rare variants; local mutation data should guide panel selection.
- If common mutations are undetected, Sanger DNA sequencing is performed at nodal centers to identify rare mutations, ensuring accuracy before proceeding to fetal testing.
- Chorionic villus sampling (CVS) is preferred over amniotic fluid for earlier (9–13 weeks) sampling, higher DNA yield, quicker results, and reduced parental anxiety.
- CVS/amniotic samples must be cleared of maternal tissue to avoid maternal cell contamination (MCC), monitored using VNTR markers such as D1S80 and APOB to ensure diagnostic accuracy.
- Once fetal DNA is obtained, parental mutations are checked via PCR ARMS to classify the fetus as unaffected, carrier, or affected, with all results reconfirmed in repeat testing.
- If the fetus is diagnosed as affected, counsellors must inform parents of implications, discuss options without directive bias, and guide decision-making compassionately.

SUGGESTED READINGS

1. Thiyagarajan A, Bhattacharya S, Sharma N, et al. Need for a universal thalassemia screening programme in India? A public health perspective. J Family Med Prim Care. 2019;8(5):1528-32.
2. Verma IC, Saxena R, Kohli S. Past, present and future scenario of thalassaemic care and control in India. Indian J Med Res. 2011;134(4):507-21.
3. Traeger-Synodinos J, Harteveld CL, Old JM, et al. EMQN best practice guidelines for molecular and haematology methods for carrier identification and prenatal diagnosis of the haemoglobinopathies. Eur J Hum Genet. 2015;23(4):426-37.
4. Vrettou C, Kakourou G, Mamas T, et al. Prenatal and preimplantation diagnosis of hemoglobinopathies. Int J Lab Hematol. 2018;40(Suppl 1):74-82.
5. Old J, Angastiniotis M, Eleftheniou A, et al. Prevention of Thalassaemias and Other Haemoglobin Disorders, 2nd edition. Nicosia: Thalassaemia International Federation; 2013. pp. 49-57.
6. Kor-anantakul O, Suwanrath C, Lutunaporn R, et al. Prenatal diagnosis of thalassemia in Songklanagarind Hospital in southern Thailand. Southeast Asian J Trop Med Public Health. 1998;29(4):795-800.
7. Kukreti R, Dash D, Vineetha KE, et al. Spectrum of β-thalassemia mutations and their association with allelic sequence polymorphisms at the β-globin gene cluster in an eastern Indian population. Am J Hematol. 2002;70(4):269-77.
8. Mohanty D, Kolah R. Laboratory Manual for Screening, Diagnosis and Molecular Analysis of Haemoglobinopathies and Red Cell Enzymopathies. Mumbai, India: Bhalani Publishing House; 2008. pp. 98-101.
9. Colah R, Gorakshakar A, Nadkarni A, et al. Regional heterogeneity of β-thalassemia mutations in the multiethnic Indian population. Blood Cells Mol Dis. 2009;42(3):241-6.
10. Dasgupta S, Chaudhury K, Mukherjee K. Usefulness of chorionic villus sampling for prenatal diagnosis of thalassaemia: a clinical study in eastern India. Int J Reprod Contracept Obstet Gynecol. 2015;4(3):790-4.
11. Thakur C, Vaz F, Banerjee M, et al. Prenatal diagnosis of β-thalassaemia and other haemoglobinopathies in India. Prenat Diagn. 2000;20(3):194-201.

8

CHAPTER

Thalassemia and Blood Transfusion

Biplabendu Talukdar, Rajendra Chaudhary

INTRODUCTION

The first blood transfusion for thalassemia patients was performed in 1925 by a Greek physician named George Papanicolaou. He transfused a 5-year-old boy with beta-thalassemia major who had severe anemia and bone deformities. The transfusion improved the boy's condition and prolonged his life for several months. A blood transfusion program is essential to managing thalassemia, a genetic disorder that produces abnormal hemoglobin. Thalassemia patients require regular blood transfusions to maintain an adequate hemoglobin level for tissue oxygenation and prevent complications associated with severe anemia. In the majority of thalassemic patients, transfusion of blood is needed from an early age. According to the transfusion requirement, thalassemia patients are classified as transfusion-dependent (TDT) and nontransfusion-dependent (NTDT). Diagnosis should be confirmed before the transfusion program starts in an individual.

KEY ASPECTS OF TRANSFUSION IN THALASSEMIC

- When and whom to transfuse.
- Frequency of transfusion
- Packed red blood cells.
- Pretransfusion testing
- Iron chelation therapy
- Transfusion monitoring
- Transfusion reactions
- Long-term complications.
- Transfusion-transmitted infection.

When and Whom to Transfuse

The criteria for initiating transfusion therapy depend on the type and severity of thalassemia, clinical manifestations, and the hemoglobin level. People with transfusion-dependent thalassemia (TDT) usually start before 2 years of age, when they become symptomatic anemia with less than 7 g/dL hemoglobin. Transfusion aims to maintain the hemoglobin level above 9.5–10.5 g/dL for TDT. The decision of transfusion in NTDT (including β-thalassemia intermedia or mild to moderate hemoglobin E/β,δβ-thalassemia) is not based on hemoglobin alone. For symptomatic patients of anemia or features of extramedullary hematopoiesis, target hemoglobin levels are maintained as per TDT until puberty is complete to improve quality of life. Progressive reduction of transfusion volume and frequency of transfusion undertaken if the patient can tolerate.

Pregnant patients with thalassemia: Pretransfusion Hb at 10 g/dL reduces maternal cardiovascular stress and helps improve fetal outcome. In NTDT patients with thalassemia who have Hb below 8 g/dL, a top-up transfusion is required at 37–38 weeks of gestation to prepare for delivery.

Frequency of Transfusion

It may vary depending on the severity and physical activity of the thalassemia patients. The primary goals of transfusions are:

- Optimal recovery of donor erythrocytes in the recipient's body.
- Maximum half-life of donor RBCs in the recipient's body
- Maintaining pretransfusion of desired Hb levels and following the checklist (CBC, TTI status, serum ferritin, growth chart, spleen size, and cardiac function)
- Avoidance of transfusion-related complications.

Optimal recovery of donor erythrocytes depends on healthy, nonremunerated, voluntary, regular blood donors.

Calculation of blood volume to be transfused:

Body weight × (Desire Hb – Recent Hb)/ Hct × 3 = volume in milliliters.

Note:

- Hematocrit is 0.65 in red cell concentration, and 3–4 mL/kg PRBCS may help with a 1 g/L Hb increment in everyone.
- In routine practice, 15–20 mL/kg of packed RBCs transfused would result in a 2–3 g/dL hemoglobin increment, assuming the bag's hematocrit is near 60%.
- Two units of PRBCs may be transfused in a single setting in patients weighing more than 30 kg and over 10 years of age, which may be cost-effective for those using a commercial leukofilter.
- For TDT patient transfusion interval every 3 weeks and NTDT patients' may transfuse every 4 weeks.

Packed Red Cells Transfusion

Devoid of plasma, platelets, and white blood cells. This helps to reduce the risk of:

- Alloimmunization, and autoimmunization **(Table 1)**
- Iron overload.
- Other transfusion-related common complications

TABLE 1: The differences between alloimmunization and autoimmunization.

	Alloimmunization	Autoimmunization
Features	Recipients have red cell antibodies against non-self-donor antigens	Recipients have red cell antibodies against the self-antigen
Frequencies	10–20% have features of alloimmunization and need chronic blood transfusion. It is more common among children being treated with a transfusion therapy after 1–3 years of age	Autoantibodies may be associated with alloantibodies. Multiple cohorts of multi-transfused patients' data revealed that approximately 8% had RBCs auto-antibodies among all antibodies
Antigens responsible	Nearly 80% have antibodies against c, C, E, and Kell antigens, and 5–10% have antibodies against other rare red cell antigens	Cold auto-antibodies against P or I antigen and warm auto-antibodies have Rh specificity
Laboratory parameters	• React only to allogenic cells, not to own cells i.e., DAT and IAT positive • Reticulocyte count. • Allo-antibody screening -3 cells followed by 11 cells • Bone marrow evaluation	• React with one's own red cells i.e., DAT, auto positive • Reticulocyte count • Allo-antibody screening cells show pan reactivity • Bone marrow evaluation
Managements	Corresponding antigen-negative red cell transfusion	Immune autoantibody treated with either steroid/IVIG/rituximab

Alloimmunization/autoimmunization suspected in case of sudden increases in transfusion frequencies due to evidence of acute or delayed hemolytic transfusion reactions.

Pretransfusion Testing

Pretransfusion testing and extended Rh and Kell phenotype-matched donor units with Coombs crossmatch with recipients' serum/plasma by donor cells minimized transfusion-related adverse events.

The following measures are essential for pretransfusion testing.

Preanalytical:

- Identification of recipients along with the phlebotomist's name
- Sample collection in an EDTA and clotted sterile vacutainer.
- A freshly collected 2 mL sample is always preferred for testing.
- All parameters must be filled in the requisition form.
- For the sample to be transported, the cold chain must be maintained.

Analytical:

- Identification of the sample
- Devoid of hemolysis
- Confirmation of blood group–preferably in two different persons
- Antibody screening and identification
- Extended Rh and Kell phenotyping with matched donor units for transfusion
- Always Coombs crossmatch by donor cells and recipients' serum
- Prestorage leukoreduced PRBCS are preferable.
- Donor units not less than 14 days old.
- For irregular antibodies in the recipient's blood, respective antigen-negative units must be transfused (depending upon the clinical significance of the antibody)

Postanalytical: Any unwanted events during and after transfusion should be recorded, and the following samples should be sent to the blood center for post-analysis.

- Respective blood bags along with transfusion sets
- Post-transfusion blood samples (EDTA, clotted)
- Post-transfusion urine sample

Note: Donor units should be transfused as early as possible, and transfusion should be completed within 4 hours from when the blood center issues the donor units.

Warming of donor units is not required until massive transfusion and neonatal transfusion (blood warmer must be used for neonatal transfusion)

Iron Chelation Therapy

It is required for transfusion-dependent thalassemic patients. The following calculation helps to determine the deposition of serum iron in everyone.

Volume of PRBC transfusion in mL × 0.47 = total iron deposition in mg

1 mL of blood contains 0.47 mg of iron.

Chelation therapy depends upon the TIF guidelines.

Note: According to the British Society of Haematology (BSH), the formula used for the calculation of iron loading mg/kg/day: Units of blood transfusion (annum) × 200/(patients weight × 365).

Transfusion Monitoring

It is one of the key management areas in the transfusion service.

- The blood bag and patients are identified simultaneously.
- Cold chain maintenance during transportation.
- Avoid storage of components apart from the blood bank refrigerator (BBR)
- Monitor transfusion-related adverse events.

- Post-transfusion Hb increment after 1/24 hours.

Transfusion Reactions

Any unwanted transfusion-related events must be reported in India's haemovigilance program.

Common transfusion reactions are given below:

- *Adverse events*: Any unintentional or undesirable occurrence before, during, or after transfusion. It may result from an error or incident, i.e., a lack of GMP or SOP.
- *Adverse reactions*: Undesirable temporary reactions to recipients by donor units following transfusion of blood or components, i.e., incorrect blood components, ABO mismatched, wrong identification, etc.

Allogenic blood transfusion-mediated adverse events are as follows **(Flowchart 1)**.

Transfusion reactions are based on their time of onset.

Onset of transfusion reactions based on timing is summarized in **Table 2**.

Common Transfusion Reaction

Table 3 summarizes the details of common transfusion reactions, including clinical features, diagnosis and management.

TABLE 2: Transfusion reactions are based on their time of onset.

Transfusion reactions within 24 hours	**Time of onset after transfusion**	**Probable cause of reaction**
	Within 1 hour	TAH
	Within 4 hours	FNHTR, allergic reaction
	Within 6/12 hours	TRALI, TACO
	Within 24 hours	HTR, TAD
Transfusion reactions after 24 hours	**Onset between**	**Probable cause of reaction**
	24 hours to 28 days	DHTR, DSTR
	5–12 days	PTP
	7–42 days	TA-GVHD

FNHTR

Febrile nonhemolytic transfusion reaction (FNHTR) is the most common type of transfusion reaction. It is a benign occurrence with symptoms that include fever but are not directly related to hemolysis (breakdown of red blood cells). It is caused by cytokine release from leukocytes (white blood cells) within the donor product because of white blood cell breakdown. These inflammatory mediators accumulate during the storage of the donated blood, so the frequency of this reaction increases with the storage length of donated blood.

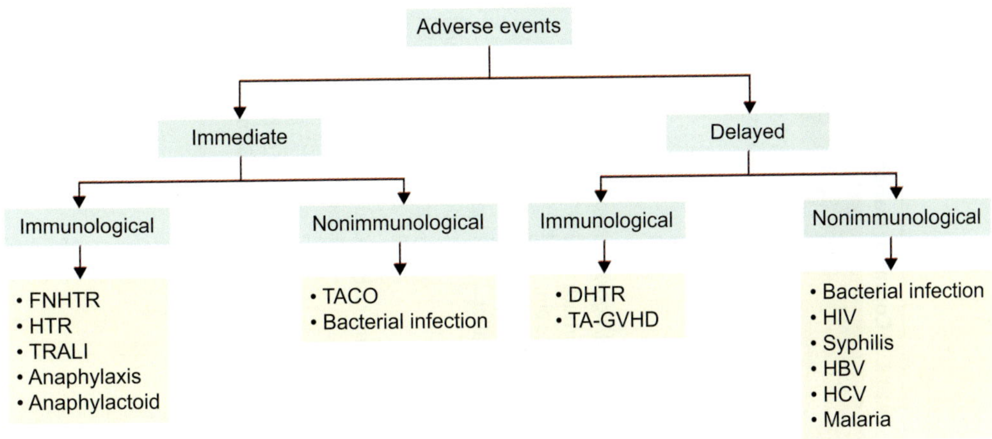

FLOWCHART 1: Allogeneic blood transfusion reactions.

TABLE 3: Common transfusion reaction.

Symptoms	Sign	Laboratory parameter	Diagnosis	Managements	Prevention	Differential diagnosis
Fever, chills/rigor, within 4 hours	Fever ≥38°C or ≥ 1°C from pretransfusion value	• DAT, IAT-negative • No urine hemoglobin • No growth in bacterial culture	FNHTR	• Discontinue transfusion • Antipyretics	Pre-storage leukoreduction	HTR Sepsis
Fever, chill/rigors chest pain/back pain/flank pain within 24 hours	Hypotension, pallor, jaundice, diffuse bleeding	DAT, IAT-positive, hemoglobinemia, hemoglobinurea	AHTR	Maintain hydration, inducing diuresis and vasodilatation, IVIG, Red cell exchange	Pretransfusion testing, antibody identification and antigen-negative blood transfusion	Sepsis
Fatigue, pallor, jaundice 2–28 days	Unexpected progressive anemia and jaundice	DAT, IAT-positive, LDH, decrease serum haptoglobin	DHTR	Maintain hydration, IVIG, red cell exchange	Proper pretransfusion testing, antibody screening, antigen negative units transfusion	DSTR
Morbilliform rash, pruritus	Caugh, wheezing, bronchospasm	Preformed IgE antibody/IgA deficiency	Allergic/ anaphylactic	Stop the the transfusion, administer antihistaminics	Washed red cells, plasma or platelet reduction	TAH
Hypotension/ facial flasing	A drop of systolic pressure 30 mm Hg	All test are negative	TAH	Cessation of transfusion, inotropic supports	Avoid bedside leucofilter. Avoid ACE inhibitors 24-48 hours before	Allergic reaction, anaphylaxis, HTR

FNHTR usually occurs during or within four hours of a transfusion. The symptoms may also include chills, rigors, increased respiratory rate, change in blood pressure, anxiety, and a headache. However, these symptoms may also occur in other more serious transfusion reactions, such as acute hemolytic reaction, transfusion-transmitted bacterial infection and transfusion-related acute lung injury (TRALI). Therefore, FNHTR is a diagnosis of exclusion and requires careful evaluation.

The treatment of FNHTR involves stopping the transfusion immediately and following other steps to manage suspected transfusion reactions. The fever can be treated with an antipyretic (fever-reducing) drug, such as paracetamol. However, aspirin should be avoided in thrombocytopenic (low platelet count) and pediatric (child) patients. If other causes of fever have been excluded, it may be possible to restart the transfusion slowly, with appropriate patient observation.

To prevent FNHTR, leukoreduction (removal of white blood cells) of future transfusions is sometimes performed. This can reduce the occurrence of this reaction by lowering the number of cytokines and leukocyte antibodies in the blood product. However, leukoreduction is not 100% effective, and some patients may still experience FNHTR despite receiving leukoreduced blood products.

Hemolytic Transfusion Reaction

A HTR is a serious complication that can occur after a blood transfusion. It happens when the red blood cells that were given during the transfusion are destroyed by the person's immune system. This can cause symptoms such as fever, chills, back pain, dark urine, and shortness of breath. It can also lead to kidney failure, shock, and death.

There are different types of hemolytic transfusion reactions, depending on the cause and timing of the response. The most common type is acute hemolytic transfusion reaction (AHTR), which occurs within 24 hours of the transfusion and can be triggered by a few milliliters of blood. AHTR is usually caused by ABO incompatibility, which means that the donor's blood type does not match the recipient's blood type. For example, if a person with type A blood receives type B, their immune system will produce antibodies against the B antigens on the donor's red blood cells and destroy them.

Another type of hemolytic transfusion reaction is called delayed hemolytic transfusion reaction (DHTR), which occurs more than 24 hours after the transfusion and can take up to several weeks to develop. Other blood group incompatibilities, such as Rh, Kell, Duffy, or Kidd, usually cause DHTR. These are minor antigens that are not routinely tested before a transfusion. A person may not have antibodies against these antigens at the time of the transfusion but may develop them later due to exposure to the donor's red blood cells.

The treatment of hemolytic transfusion reactions depends on the severity and type of the response. The first step is to stop the transfusion immediately and notify the blood bank. The blood samples from the recipient and the donor should be tested to confirm the diagnosis and identify the cause of the reaction. The recipient should be monitored closely for signs of hemolysis, kidney damage, and shock. They may need supportive care such as fluids, oxygen, blood pressure medications, and dialysis. They may also need medications to remove excess iron from the body or to prevent further antibody production.

To prevent hemolytic transfusion reactions, it is essential to follow strict protocols for blood typing and cross-matching before a transfusion. Blood banks should screen donated blood for infectious agents and common antigens. Recipients should be informed of their blood type and any previous transfusions or pregnancies that may have sensitized them to specific antigens. They should also be educated about the signs and symptoms of a transfusion reaction and instructed to report them immediately if they occur.

Pulmonary Adverse Events

The common pulmonary adverse events include TRALI and TACO **(Table 4)**.

Transfusion-related Acute Lung Injury

Transfusion-related acute lung injury is a serious and potentially fatal complication of blood transfusion that causes fluid to accumulate in the lungs and impair oxygen delivery. Here are some key points about TRALI:

TRALI usually occurs within 6 hours of receiving a blood product, especially those containing plasma. Immune or nonimmune mechanisms can cause TRALI. Immune-mediated TRALI involves antibodies from the donor that react with the recipient's white blood cells or lung cells. Nonimmune-mediated TRALI involves bioactive lipids from the stored blood that activate the recipient's white blood cells. TRALI can present with symptoms such as fever, chills, shortness of breath, low blood pressure, and low oxygen levels. It can be difficult to distinguish from other causes of lung injury, such as infection or fluid overload. TRALI is diagnosed by excluding other possible causes and by testing the donor and recipient blood for antibodies. It is treated by stopping the transfusion, providing oxygen and supportive care, and monitoring the patient closely. TRALI can be prevented by reducing the use of plasma products, screening donors for antibodies, and removing white blood cells from blood products.

Anaphylaxis

Transfusion-related anaphylaxis is a rare but severe allergic reaction that can occur after receiving a blood product, especially those containing plasma. It is characterized by a systemic life-threatening response, typically presenting as bronchospasm, respiratory distress, and hypotension. It can be caused by different mechanisms, such as:

- Anti-IgA antibodies in the recipient react with IgA in the donor plasma. This is more common in patients with IgA deficiency.
- Performed antibodies in the recipient against allergens, drugs, or chemicals in the donor plasma.
- Nonimmune-mediated activation of mast cells and basophils by bioactive substances in the stored blood product.

The treatment of transfusion-related anaphylaxis involves stopping the transfusion immediately and following the steps for managing suspected transfusion reactions. The patient should receive oxygen, intravenous fluids, epinephrine, antihistamines, and corticosteroids as needed. The blood samples from the donor and recipient should be tested for antibodies

TABLE 4: Pulmonary adverse events.

Symptoms	Sign	Laboratory testing	Diagnosis	Management	Prevention
Hypoxemia, tachycardia respiratory distress within 6 hours	BP normal or low, pulse pressure normal	CXR-white lung field, no pleural fluid. SpO_2 <90%,	TRALI	Oxygen therapy, mechanical ventilation	Avoid plasma-rich products from multigravida
Shortness of breath, cough, tachycardia	Increase BP, widened pulse pressure	White lung fields increase the cardiac silhouette. Pleural fluid	TACO	Diuretics, phlebotomy	Avoid multiple-unit transfusions

and other reaction causes. The transfusion service should be notified, and the reaction should be reported to the hemovigilance system.

To prevent transfusion-related anaphylaxis, some strategies include:

- Screening donors for IgA deficiency and anti-IgA antibodies.
- Using washed red blood cells or platelets to remove plasma and other substances.
- Using solvent-detergent-treated plasma or pathogen-reduced plasma to inactivate antibodies and other agents.
- Using IgA-depleted or IgA-deficient plasma for patients with Iga deficiency.

Other transfusion-related complications are given below:

- Anaphylactoid reaction
- Metabolic complications (hypocalcemia, hyperkalemia, and hypokalemia)
- TA-GVHD (transfusion-associated graft vs. host disease)
- PTP (post-transfusion purpura)
- TRIM (transfusion-related immuno-modulation)
- Bacterial infection
- Viral infections

Long-term Complications

While blood transfusions are a lifesaving treatment for thalassemia, they can lead to certain long-term complications, as given below.

- Iron overload in various organs, including the heart, liver, and endocrine glands
- Organ dysfunctions, heart failure, arrhythmia, cardiomyopathy, and liver cirrhosis
- Endocrine abnormalities followed by diabetes, hypothyroidism, and delayed puberty in children
- Viral infections
- Allo- and autoimmunization

It is important to note that the specific details of the transfusion program can vary depending on the patients' condition and the protocols followed by the treating medical team. Therefore, thalassemia patients need to receive care from a specialized healthcare provider experienced in managing the disorder.

Transfusion-transmitted Infections

Common pathogens can be transmitted through a donor's blood transfusion to recipients **(Table 5)**.

CONCLUSION

Transfusions help maintain target hemoglobin levels (typically 9.5–10.5 g/dL for β-thalassemia major) to support normal growth, prevent fatigue, and avoid complications. Most older children and adults receive transfusions every 3 weeks, while younger children and those with HbE β-thalassemia may receive them every 4 weeks. Patients with thalassemia intermedia who start transfusions later in life face higher risks of alloimmunization and hemolytic transfusion reactions. Long-term transfusions lead to iron accumulation, requiring iron chelation therapy to prevent organ damage. Factors such as spleen status, weight, heart function, and fatigue influence transfusion strategies.

SUMMARY

- Regular blood transfusions are a cornerstone of managing transfusion-dependent thalassemia (TDT), aiming to maintain hemoglobin levels at 9.5–10.5 g/dL to ensure optimal oxygen delivery and prevent anemia-related complications.
- Transfusion initiation depends on severity, type of thalassemia, and associated symptoms; TDT patients often start before age 2, while NTDT patients receive transfusions for symptomatic anemia or extramedullary hematopoiesis.

TABLE 5: Common transfusion transmitted infections.

Pathogen	Types	C/F	Laboratory investigation	Remarks
Viruses	HIV 1 and 2	Flu-like symptoms, myalgia, skin rash, anorexia, unexplained diarrhea, increased transfusion, etc.	• Rapid testing • ELISA • CLI	Refer to ICTC followed by ART clinic
	Hepatitis A	Fever, Jaundice, anorexia	Anti-HAV IgM and IgG antibodies	Refer to medicine or hepatology
	Hepatitis B	Fever, Jaundice,	HBsAg, Anti-HBc testing, HBV-DNA by NAT testing	Refer to hepatology or NVHCP
	Hepatitis C	Fever, Jaundice, increased transfusion, etc.	• Anti-HCV by ELISA/CLI • HCV-RNA by NAT testing	Refer to hepatology following the NVHCP protocol
	Hepatitis E	Fever, malaise, anorexia, jaundice	Anti-HbE IgM or IgG	Refer to hepatology
Parasites	Plasmodium	Post-transfusion history of fever with diurnal variation	Thick and thin blood smear of peripheral blood, IFTA/ELISA, NAT test	Refer to medicine for anti-plasmodium treatment
Spirochaete	Treponema	Non-specific	Gram-negative rod or spirochaete. TPHA	Refer to STI clinic for further management

- Packed red blood cells (PRBCs) are preferred for transfusion as they reduce plasma and leukocyte-mediated complications, including alloimmunization and autoimmunization.
- Transfusion intervals typically follow every 3 weeks for TDT and every 4 weeks for NTDT, with transfusion volumes calculated based on body weight, Hb targets, and PRBC hematocrit values.
- Extended Rh and Kell antigen matching, Coombs crossmatching, and prestorage leukoreduction reduce immune reactions; meticulous pre-, intra-, and post-transfusion procedures are essential for safety.
- Transfusion reactions range from febrile nonhemolytic to acute or delayed hemolytic reactions, allergic responses, hypotension (TAH), and pulmonary complications such as TRALI and TACO.
- Transfusion-transmitted infections, including HIV, hepatitis viruses, malaria, and syphilis, must be screened and managed per national guidelines.
- Iron overload is a major long-term risk, requiring chelation therapy guided by transfusion frequency and iron loading formulas from TIF or BSH guidelines.
- Monitoring includes post-transfusion Hb increments, vigilance for adverse events, and hemovigilance reporting to India's national program.
- Special considerations apply to pregnant women with thalassemia, ensuring Hb ≥10 g/dL predelivery, and to older NTDT patients, who face increased alloimmunization risks.

SUGGESTED READINGS

1. Ministry of Health and Family Welfare. Transfusion Medicine technical manual, 3rd edition, revised in 2023, New Delhi: Ministry of Health and Family Welfare; 2023.
2. Indian Academy of Paediatrics. Evidence-based IAP-PHO Guidelines for Diagnosis and Management of Thalassemia-2023, 1st edition. India: Indian Academy of Paediatrics; 2023.
3. Simon TL, McCullough J, Snyder EL, et al. Rossi's Textbook of Transfusion Medicine, 5th edition. Philadelphia: Wiley-Blackwell; 2016.
4. Cappellini MD, Cohen A, Porter J, et al. Guidelines for managing Transfusion dependent thalassemia (TDT), 3rd edition. Nicosia (CY): Thalassaemia International Federation; 2014.
5. Hillyer CD, Silberstein LE, Ness PM, et al. Blood banking and transfusion medicine: Basic principles and practice. Philadelphia: Elsevier Health Sciences; 2006.

9

CHAPTER

Iron Overload in Thalassemia—Diagnosis and Management

Rajib De, Chirasree Sanyal

INTRODUCTION

Iron overload is an inevitable consequence in both transfusion-dependent thalassemia (TDT) and nontransfusion-dependent thalassemia (NTDT). The main sources of iron overload is either RBC transfusion and/or increased GI absorption, in view of ineffective erythropoiesis. Iron overload can damage vital organs such as the heart, liver, and endocrine glands. Effective management of iron overload is crucial for both groups to improve patient outcomes and prevent complications.

IRON HOMEOSTASIS AND PATHOPHYSIOLOGY OF IRON OVERLOAD

The majority of iron required for erythropoiesis (90–95%) is recycled from senescent RBCs by reticuloendothelial macrophages. Transferrin binds iron after undergoing a conformational change and forms nontoxic transferrin-bound iron (TBI) and is usually around 30% saturated. When transferrin saturation exceeds 70%, non-transferrin-bound iron (NTBI) accumulates and produces reactive oxygen species, causing target organ damage **(Fig. 1)**.

- Increased GI absorption
- Occasional blood transfusion **(Fig. 2)**

Organ Affected

Liver

The liver is the primary organ affected by oxidative stress due to iron overload. Key impacts include:

- Liver fibrosis/cirrhosis
- Hepatocellular carcinoma

Heart

Cardiac damage includes:

- Cardiac siderosis
- Heart failure
- Pulmonary hypertension

Endocrine System

Iron overload contributes to various endocrine dysfunctions, including hypothyroidism, hypoparathyroidism, growth retardation, hypogonadotropic hypogonadism, osteoporosis, and diabetes mellitus.

MONITORING IRON OVERLOAD

Multiple diagnostic tests are available for assessing iron overload. Their interpretation often requires specialized expertise.

Diagnostic Approaches

Invasive Methods

Liver biopsy: Historically the gold standard but now largely replaced by noninvasive techniques.

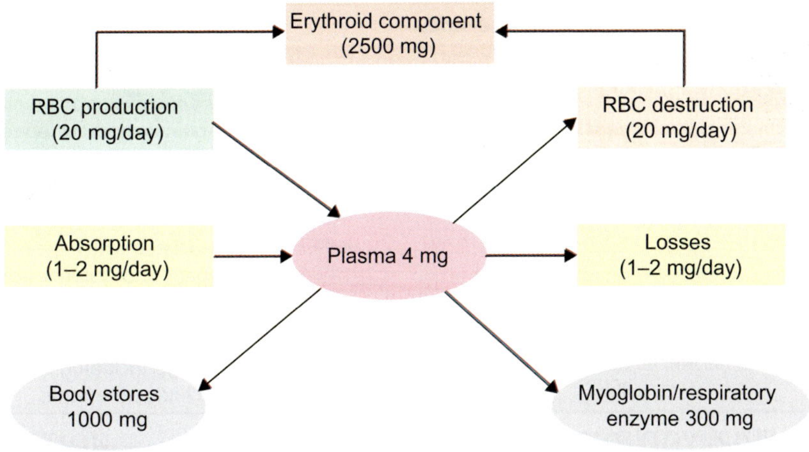

FIG. 1: Pathophysiology of iron overload.

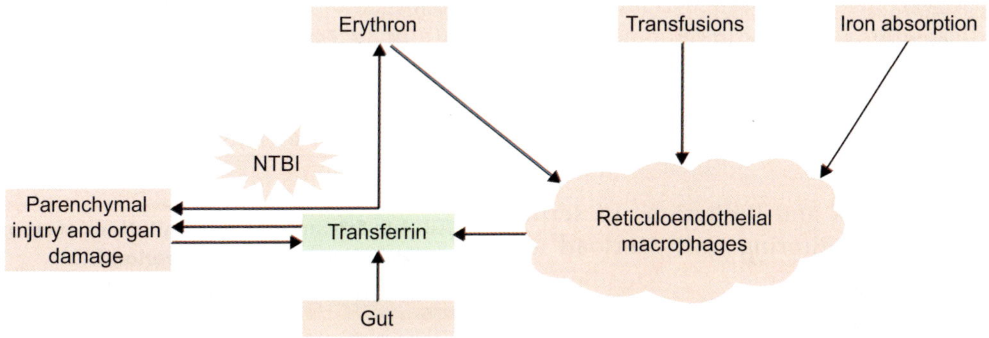

FIG. 2: Causes of iron overload in TDT and NTDT.

(NTDT: nontransfusion-dependent thalassemia; TDT: transfusion-dependent thalassemia)

Noninvasive Methods

- *Serum ferritin*: The most used, cost-effective marker, but its levels are influenced by inflammation and liver injury.
- *T2* MRI (liver/heart)*: The gold standard for detecting iron overload in specific organs.
- *24-hour urinary iron estimation*: Measures iron excretion following chelation therapy. Not necessary in routine use.

Classification according to iron overload severity is shown in **Table 1**.[1]

Liver

- LIC measured by T2* MRI provides most reliable estimate of total body iron
- Total body iron stores in mg iron/kg body weight = 10.6 × the LIC (in mg/g dry weight)
- LIC and serum ferritin may not always be linear.

Cardiac T2* MRI values and their clinical significance are shown in **Table 2**.[2]

Risk of developing heart failure associated with 160 folds higher in the next year of TDT with T2* values < 6 ms.[3]

TABLE 1: Classification of iron overload severity.

Severity	Liver iron concentration (LIC) (mg/g dry weight)	Serum ferritin range (µg/L)	Transferrin saturation (TSAT)(%)	Clinical notes
Mild	3–7	300–500 (men) 200–300 (women)	>45%	Typically asymptomatic; requires monitoring to prevent progression of iron overload
Moderate	7–15	500–1000	>60%	Associated with increasing risk of hepatic and systemic iron-related complications
Severe	>15	>1000 or clinically significant elevation	>80%	Strongly linked to end-organ damage, including cardiac, hepatic, and endocrine issues

TABLE 2: Risk categories for cardiac iron overload by MRI.

Risk category	Cardiac T2* (ms)	Clinical significance
Low risk	>20 ms	Indicates minimal or no cardiac iron deposition; very low probability of cardiac dysfunction
Intermediate risk	10–20 ms	Suggests moderate myocardial iron accumulation; associated with a greater chance of cardiac performance abnormalities
High risk	<10 ms	Reflects substantial cardiac iron burden; strongly correlated with increased chances of heart failure and rhythm disturbances

Advantages and limitations of serum ferritin in monitoring iron overload are shown in **Table 3**.

Suggested Monitoring Methods

- The recommended method for monitoring iron overload is ferritin in all OPD.
- Monitoring for ferritin to be started after 2 years of age or after >10 units of blood transfusion in cases of TDT.[4]
- Monitoring is to be started for all NTDT patients >5 years of age.[5]
- All patients may be screened by T2* MRI after age of > 5 years annually or every 2 years; they can be referred to higher centers for this test.

Monitoring schedules for TDT and NTDT are presented in **Table 4.**[4,5]

TABLE 3: Advantages and limitations of serum ferritin in monitoring iron overload.

Advantages	Disadvantages
• Easy to assess repeatedly • Inexpensive • Repeated estimation identifies the trend • Long term control linked to outcome • Useful for dose adjustment	• Ferritin level increased in inflammation and hepatitis and/or liver injury • In NTDT serum ferritin tends to underestimate body iron storage • Indirect estimate of iron burden • Mostly non-linear response with high iron overload • Absence of decrease doesn't exclude response • Relationship to iron load varies with chelator • Relationship to LIC differs in different types of thalassemia

CHELATION THERAPY

Chelation therapy aims to remove excess iron and prevent organ damage. The choice

TABLE 4: Recommended monitoring methods for assessing iron overload in TDT and NTDT.

Time point	TDT (transfusion-dependent thalassemia)	NTDT (non-transfusion-dependent thalassemia)
Initial (Baseline)	• Check serum ferritin • Perform liver MRI to assess LIC • Conduct cardiac T2* MRI	• Check serum ferritin • Perform liver MRI to assess LIC
Every 3 months	Monitor serum ferritin	Monitor serum ferritin
Annually	• Monitor serum ferritin • Repeat liver MRI for LIC • Repeat cardiac T2* MRI	• Monitor serum ferritin • Repeat liver MRI for LIC

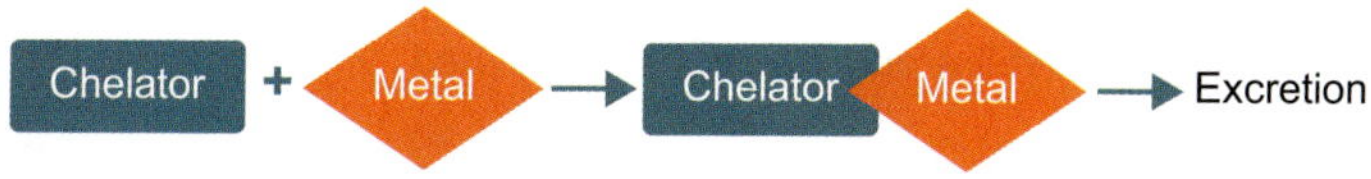

FIG. 3: Mechanism of chelation.

of chelation depends on iron burden, patient compliance, and organ involvement. The mechanism is illustrated in **Figure 3**.

When to Start Chelation

TDT:

- 2 years of age or older
- Blood transfusion > 10 units[4]
- Serum ferritin > 1,000 μg/L
- TDT patients < 2 years of age requiring chelation therapy to be referred to a higher center

NTDT:

- 5 years of age or older
- Serum ferritin level ≥ 800 μg/L
- Liver iron concentration ≥5 mg Fe/g dry weight (If facility available)

When to Discontinue

TDT:

- To reduce the dose of chelation therapy if ferritin < 500 μg/L[6]
- To discontinue chelation if LIC< 3 mg/g dry weight and/or ferritin < 300 μg/L

NTDT:

- To reduce the dose of chelation therapy if ferritin < 500 μg/L
- To discontinue chelation if LIC < 3 g/g dry weight and/or ferritin < 300 μg/L
- Pregnancy

Chelating Agents

A comparison of major iron chelators is shown in **Table 5**.

Vitamin C may be considered with standard regimen—1–2 mg/kg/day cautiously. More than 2–3 mg/kg/day as a supplement are not recommended, taken at the time of the DFO infusion for rapid chelation.

Combined or Sequential Chelator Treatment

When two different iron chelators are administered on the same day for a synergistic effect, the regimen is called combined or associated treatment, while if administered on different days, it is then referred to as alternating or sequential treatment. Studies have shown that use of sequential iron chelation with deferoxamine (DFO) and deferiprone (DFP) or DFO and deferasirox (DFX) or DFX and DFP has a significant effect on the serum ferritin and LIC.

TABLE 5: Chelating agents with route of administration, common adverse effects, and contraindications.

Parameter	Deferoxamine (DFO)	Deferiprone (DFP)	Deferasirox (DFX)
Chelator type	Hexadentate	Bidentate	Tridentate
Typical dose	20–60 mg/kg/day (max 40 mg/kg/day in children). In heart failure: Continuous 24 hours infusion with 50–60 mg/kg/day	75–100 mg/kg/day	20–40 mg/kg/day; film-coated tablet (FCT) approx imately 0.7 × dispersible tablet dose
Administration route	Subcutaneous or intravenous	Oral	Oral
Half-life	About 20–30 minutes	2–3 hours	8–16 hours
Frequency	Infused over 8–10 hours per session, 5–7 times/week	Three times daily	Once daily
Use in children (2–6 years)	Preferred first-line option	Not advised	First-line choice
Use in children >6 years and adults	First-line therapy	Used when other chelators are not tolerated or ineffective	First-line therapy
Primary route of excretion	Urine and feces	Primarily urinary	Mainly fecal
Common adverse effects	Hearing or vision issues, growth concerns, bone changes, skin discoloration, infection risk (Yersinia, viral)	Severe neutropenia, agranulocytosis, arthritis, digestive upset	Rash, abdominal discomfort, impaired kidney function
Contraindications	Pregnancy (third trimester), known allergy	Pregnancy, prior neutropenia, hypersensitivity	Pregnancy, hypersensitivity, low kidney function (GFR <60 mL/min), hepatic or renal disease

Criteria for initiation, dose reduction, and discontinuation are summarized in **Table 6**.

Monitoring of Chelation

Monitoring schedules for chelation therapy are shown in **Table 7**.

Thresholds for Concern[7]

- *Renal function*:
    - *Serum creatinine >1.2 mg/dL*: Baseline serum creatinine levels above this value were criteria for exclusion, indicating potential renal impairment.
    - *Serum creatinine > 2 mg/dL*: An increase to this level may signify acute renal failure, necessitating immediate cessation of chelation therapy.
- *Liver function tests*:
    - *SGOT/SGPT > 4 × ULN*: Patients with baseline SGOT or SGPT levels exceeding four times the ULN (i.e., > 160 IU/L) were excluded from certain studies due to increased risk of hepatotoxicity.
    - *SGOT/SGPT > 5 × ULN*: Elevations beyond five times the ULN (i.e., > 200 IU/L) are generally considered significant and may warrant discontinuation of therapy.

Conditions when a patient is to be referred to the higher center/ICSH:

- Patients with NTDT and suspected iron overload with disproportionately low ferritin should be referred to a nodal center for T2* MRI for LIC.

TABLE 6: Criteria for initiation, reduction, and discontinuation of chelation in TDT and NTDT.

	TDT	NTDT
Indication to initiate IC	serum ferritin ≥1000 µg/L or LIC ≥3 mg/g dry weight liver	SF ≥800 ng/mL and/or LIC ≥5 mg/g dry weight liver
Indication for combination IC	• Serum ferritin ≥2500 µg/L and/or LIC >7 mg/g dry weight liver and/or Cardiac T2* <20 m/s • Inadequate response with 6 months of monotherapy (SF >1,500 ng/mL, LIC > 7 mg/g dry weight • Abnormal cardiac function	• LIC > 7 mg/g dry weight liver or SF >2500 µg/L • Inadequate response with 6 months of monotherapy (SF >1,500 ng/mL, LIC > 7 mg/g dry weight • Abnormal cardiac function
Indication to stop IC	Serum ferritin <300 µg/L and/or LIC < 3 mg/g dry weight liver	SF< 300 µg/L and/or LIC< 3 mg/g dry weight liver

(TDT: transfusion-dependent thalassemia; NTDT: non-transfusion dependent thalassemia; IC: iron chelation; SF: serum ferritin; LIC: liver iron concentration)

TABLE 7: Monitoring parameters and adverse-effect profile of major iron chelators.

Parameter	Deferoxamine (DFO)	Deferasirox (DFX)	Deferiprone (DFP)
General clinical review	Monthly	Monthly	Monthly
Complete blood count (ANC)	Not routinely required	Weekly for the first month, then monthly	Weekly for the first month, then monthly
Liver function tests (LFTs)	Not routinely required	Monthly	Every 3 months
Serum creatinine	Every 3 months	Monthly	Every 3 months
Eye examination	Once a year	Once a year	Once a year
Hearing evaluation (Audiogram)	Annually	Annually	Annually
Cardiac/Liver T2* MRI	Begin after 10 years of age; then every 2 years	Begin after 10 years of age; then every 2 years	Begin after 10 years of age; then every 2 years

- Patients with high ferritin value and deteriorating cardiac function—refer to higher center for T2* MRI
- TDT patients < 2 years of age requiring chelation therapy
- For any patient with inadequate response to chelation
- For starting second or third-line chelating agent
- For starting combination of chelating agents
- For persistent toxicity of chelating agent

CONCLUSION

Iron overload remains a key determinant of morbidity and mortality in thalassemia. Advances in T2* MRI and the availability of effective chelators have enabled tailored management. Deferasirox is the preferred first-line agent, while deferiprone and deferoxamine are valuable in cardiac siderosis and combination therapy. Regular monitoring and strict adherence are essential for sustained long-term outcomes.

RECOMMENDATION

Effective iron overload management requires preventive, rescue, and emergency chelation strategies to prevent complications and improve patient outcomes. Emerging therapies offer hope for better treatment options in the future.

SUMMARY

- *Chelation therapy* plays a pivotal role in preventing organ damage in thalassemia patients with iron overload. Treatment must be individualized, considering factors such as iron levels, organ involvement, and the patient's ability to adhere to therapy.
- Chelation plans should be customized based on patient/family preferences, side effect profiles, and the patient's lifestyle.
- *Deferasirox (DFX)* is currently the first-line chelation agent of choice.
- As a once-daily oral chelator, *deferasirox* is particularly effective for managing both hepatic and cardiac iron overload. Dosing should be guided by trends in serum ferritin and liver iron concentration (LIC) to avoid excessive chelation.
- *Deferoxamine (DFO)* remains highly effective, especially in cases of severe iron accumulation. It is delivered via subcutaneous/IV infusion over 8–10 hours for 5–7 days a week and demands strong treatment adherence.
- *Deferiprone (DFP)* is the most efficient agent for reducing cardiac iron levels. It is taken three times daily and requires frequent monitoring due to risks such as agranulocytosis.
- In situations where deferasirox leads to serious toxicity and the patient is older than six years, *deferiprone* may be used as a second-line option.
- *Combination therapy* using *DFO and DFP* is advised in patients with abnormal heart function, unsatisfactory response to single-agent therapy, LIC >15 mg/g dry weight, or serum ferritin >2500 μg/L.
- In this dual regimen, DFO is typically given on weekends (twice a week), while DFP is administered daily at a standard dose of 75 mg/kg/day.
- An alternative combination involves *DFX* at 20–40 mg/kg/day (7 days a week) and *DFO* at 40 mg/kg/day for 5 days per week.
- Monitoring of iron status should include serum ferritin levels, LIC, and *cardiac T2** MRI. A T2* value below 10 milliseconds is associated with high risk of cardiac failure and necessitates urgent adjustment of chelation therapy.
- Initiation of chelation in transfusion-dependent thalassemia (TDT) is recommended when LIC exceeds 7 mg/g dry weight or serum ferritin surpasses 1,000 μg/L. In nontransfusion-dependent thalassemia (NTDT), therapy should start at lower thresholds: LIC > 5 mg/g or ferritin >800 μg/L.
- Routine monitoring during therapy should assess renal function (creatinine, proteinuria), liver enzymes (ALT), neutrophil counts in those on DFP, and annual vision and hearing tests to detect DFO-related toxicity.
- *Overchelation* may lead to increased adverse effects; therefore, chelator doses should be adjusted downward as ferritin or LIC levels decline.
- Continuous surveillance is essential to identify and manage adverse events, including dose modifications or temporary therapy interruptions.
- Long-term success with chelation therapy depends on patient adherence, which can be improved through targeted education, emotional support, and addressing barriers to compliance.

REFERENCES

1. Piperno A. Classification and diagnosis of iron overload. Haematologica. 1998;83(5):447-55.
2. Kirk P, Roughton M, Porter JB, et al. Cardiac T2* MRI for cardiac risk in thalassemia major. Circulation. 2009;120(20):1961-8.
3. Taher AT, Farmakis D, Porter JB, et al. Guidelines for the Management of Transfusion-dependent Thalassaemia. Cyprus: Thalassaemia International Federation; 2025.
4. Shah FT, Porter JB, Sadasivam N, et al. Guidelines for the monitoring and management of iron overload in patients with haemoglobinopathies and rare anaemias. Br J Haematol. 2022;196(2):336-50.
5. aHuang Y, Yang G, Wang M, et al. Iron overload status in patients with non-transfusion-dependent thalassemia in China. Ther Adv Hematol. 2022;13:20406207221084639.
6. Scaramellini N, Arighi C, Marcon A, Consonni D, Cassinerio E, Graziadei G, Cappellini MD, Motta I. Iron chelation and ferritin below 500 µg/L in transfusion-dependent thalassemia: beyond the limits of clinical trials. Blood. 2019;134(Suppl 1):3542. doi:10.1182/blood-2019-130237
7. Dhamija M, Mahajan A, Kalra M, et al. Deferasirox in Indian children with thalassemia. Indian J Med Paediatr Oncol. 2013;34(1):16-20.

10
CHAPTER

Monitoring of Thalassemia Patients

Tuphan Kanti Dolai, Shipla Roy

INTRODUCTION

Thalassemia refers to a group of inherited autosomal recessive hematological diseases characterized by decreased or absent synthesis of one or more of the normal globin chains. The primary quantitative defects are now no longer differentiated from structural variants produced at a reduced rate (e.g., Hb E and Hb Lepore). Homozygotes, compound heterozygotes as well as interaction of thalassemia with corresponding hemoglobinopathies like HbE, HbC, and HbS result in thalassemia syndrome.[1-3]

Transfusion-dependent thalassemia (TDT) and nontransfusion-dependent thalassemia (NTDT) are associated with several morbidity as well as mortality if not treated adequately. It is essential to monitor the complications of both the disorders. TDT and NTDT result in iron overload in endocrine organs, heart and liver and therefore, monitoring is essential.[4] The two clinical phenotypes are distinct entities and managed in different ways. So, monitoring is the essential component of their course of illness and treatment.

MANAGEMENT AND MONITORING OF PATIENTS

Indications of Blood Transfusion[5]

- Confirmed case of thalassemia
- Hb value <7 g/dL in two consecutive occasions detected at least 2 weeks apart (excluding other contributory factors like infection)
- *Clinical criteria irrespective of Hb level:*
    - Significant symptomatic anemia
    - Poor growth or failure to thrive
    - Complications from intramedullary hematopoiesis like pathological fractures and bony changes
    - Clinically significant extramedullary hematopoiesis

Recommendation

- Extended RBC antigen typing before first transfusion at least D, C, c, E, e, and Kell
- Leukodepleted fresh packed RBC within 1 week (stored in CPD-A) and within 2 weeks (stored in additive solution) to maintain pretransfusion Hb 9.5–10.5 g/dL and post-transfusion Hb below 13–15 g/dL
- Keep a record of any history of alloimmunization and annual transfusion requirement

Monitor the Complications of Blood Transfusion

- Febrile nonhemolytic transfusion reaction-in each transfusion
- Transfusion-transmitted infection (most common is hepatitis B and C virus) every 3 months

- Iron overload-related comorbidities and complications
- Alloimmunization (most common in nontransfusion dependent and minimally transfused individuals)—monitoring clinically when suspected

Monitoring of Iron Overload

- *Serum ferritin*:
  - Serum ferritin generally correlates with body iron stores
  - Relatively easy and inexpensive to determine repeatedly
  - Value ≥ 1,000 ng/mL for TDT and 800 ng/mL for NTDT are indications of chelation therapy
  - A serum ferritin value less than 300 ng/mL is an indication of stoppage of chelation therapy
  - A sudden unexpected rise of serum ferritin may indicate hepatitis infection or other systemic infections
  - Long-term control of iron overload is linked to outcome
  - Useful for dose adjustment as iron levels fall
  - The monitoring interval is 3 months
  - Must be done before splenectomy as well as before allogeneic stem cell transplant
- *Liver iron concentration (LIC)*:
  - *Biopsy*:
    - Not routinely performed as it is invasive and can't determine if LIC is more than 30 mg/g dry weight
    - This can be done during splenectomy
    - Value > 7 mg/g dry weight for TDT and 5 mg/g dry weight for NTDT warrants iron chelation therapy
    - Persistent high LIC >15 mg/g dry weight denotes a worsened prognosis with progressive liver fibrosis
    - If LIC ranges 3–7 mg/g dry weight monitor 1–2 yearly but if > 7 mg/g dry weight, then yearly monitoring
  - *SQUID (superconducting quantum interference device)*: Uses paramagnetism technology to determine the proportion of LIC if available
  - *MRI (T2* technique)*:[6]
    - The most widely used methods for LIC determination nowadays
    - Underestimate LIC by 2–3 folds
    - Sensitivity of >85% and specificity of >92% up to a LIC of 15 mg/g dry weight
    - Noninvasive with good patient acceptance
- *Myocardial iron monitoring:*[7] Regular cardiovascular monitoring should be performed on an annual basis in all thalassemia patients. The frequency and content should be tailored to meet each patient's needs and shorter intervals (e.g., 3 or 6 monthly).
  - *Echocardiography*: Sequential monitoring of LVEF to diagnose impending heart failure
  - *MRI:*[7]
    - Myocardial T2* by MRI can identify high-risk patients before declining LVEF and has additional predictive value
    - T2* values less than 20 ms denote low LVEF
    - The risk of developing heart failure increases if T2* <10 ms
    - Can measure iron content in septum and monitor heart function simultaneously
    - If T2* >20 ms monitor 2 yearly and if 10–19 ms then monitor yearly
  - *Echocardiographic TRV (tricuspid regurgitation velocity)*:
    - Value >3.2 m/s indicates pulmonary hypertension
    - If value is < 2.5 m/s monitor 3–5 yearly

Systemic Monitoring[8-12]

- Tanner staging (10–17 years of age) annually
- Standing and sitting height every 6 months
- Growth monitoring every 3 months as per WHO scale
- Screening for HCV and HBV chronic infection is recommended in thalassemic patients every 3 monthly
- Anti HbsAb titer detection before hepatitis B vaccination
- HBV DNA and HCV-RNA load if HBsAg and anti HCV Ab detected
- Biannual ultrasound abdomen for detection of hepatic parenchymal disease
- FT4, TSH, GH, FSH, LH every yearly after 11 years of age
- Serum calcium, vitamin D3, and phosphate annually
- LFT, urea, and creatinine every 3 monthly
- FBS, PPBS, parathormone annually
- If in NTDT patients a sudden rise in ALT, or AST happens monitor HAV and HEV antibody
- X-ray of wrist and hand, tibia, and spine who have body disproportion to exclude the presence of platylospondylosis or metaphyseal cartilaginous dysplasia changes
- MRI brain to see the pituitary gland structure if indicated
- Dual energy X-ray absorptiometry (DXA) is a noninvasive technique performed on the hip, lumbar spine, and distal radius for the measurement of BMD from adolescence on yearly interval. BMD T-score ≤2.5 predicts high risk of fracture and osteopenia if BMD T-score between -1 and -2.5, with normal values of T-score being ≥1.0

Monitoring of Iron Chelation Therapy[13]

- Dose reductions guided by calculating therapeutic index [= mean daily dose (mg/kg)/serum ferritin μg/L] to keep this < 0.025
- Monitor audiometry regularly, particularly as ferritin falls
- Monitor eyes regularly including electroretinography if on high doses
- If fever occurs blood culture should be taken after hospitalization and special attention to be given for *Klebsiella, Yersinia, Pseudomonas* infection
- Always check absolute neutrophil count (ANC) before starting deferiprone therapy
- *For neutropenia*: ANC <1.5 × 109 /L interrupt treatment during deferiprone therapy
- For agranulocytosis (ANC < 1.5 × 109 /L), consider hospitalization deferiprone therapy
- Monitor for symptoms of arthropathy during deferiprone therapy
- Monitor creatinine level weekly for first 4 weeks after starting as well as dose escalation and then monthly
- LFT, urea, and creatinine every 3 monthly

Monitoring of Conception[14]

- In case of suspected infertility FT4, TSH, GH, LH, FSH, parathormone, USG lower abdomen to see the development of ovarian follicle
- Monitoring of menstrual cycle by serial vaginal ultrasound and estradiol measurement
- Baseline testosterone and semen analysis in male
- Monitoring testosterone level in each month after hCG administration
- Test for hemoglobinopathy of a spouse (CBC, PBS, reticulocyte count, ferritin, iron, Hb HPLC)
- Prenatal testing for preimplantation diagnosis as well as identifying unaffected HLA matched siblings for cord blood banking

Monitoring in Splenectomized Patients[15]

- CBC with peripheral blood smear to monitor platelet count at least 3 monthly
- TRV monitoring annually
- RBC also Ab panel if clinically indicated
- PT, INR, APTT, D dimer, USG Doppler if suspected venous thromboembolism

Monitoring in Case of Allogenic Hematopoietic Stem Cell Transplant[16]

- HLA typing for all thalassemic patients (<17 years of age) who require chronic blood transfusion with or without features of iron overload with siblings and family members
- Serum ferritin, LFT, urea, creatinine every 3 months for monitoring of iron chelation

Monitoring in Nontransfusion-dependent Thalassemia

NTDT refers to patients who do not require lifelong regular blood transfusions for survival like beta thalassemia intermedia and E beta thalassemia. Incidence of pulmonary hypertension, venous thromboembolism in splenectomized patients, extramedullary hematopoiesis is more.

- All patients more than 10 years of age should be frequently assessed for iron overload as like TDT
- Tanner staging (10–17 years of age) annually
- Standing and sitting height every 6 months
- CBC with peripheral blood smear for platelet count and nRBC strongly related to pulmonary hypertension and thromboembolic events
- Serum ferritin > 800 ng/mL indicates iron chelation requirement
- LFT, urea creatinine in every 3 months
- USG abdomen annually if LIC > 5 mg/g dry weight and serum ferritin > 800 ng/mL
- Alfa fetoprotein annually if patient is cirrhotic or age is >40 years
- Transient elastography monitoring every 12–24 months if available
- Extended RBC antigen phenotype and RBC allo-Ab panel to rule out alloimmunization
- Spine imaging by MRI if back pain and any neurological complains to exclude extramedullary hematopoiesis
- Biopsy with cytochemical stain from extramedullary hematopoietic pseudotumor
- DXA scan every 2 years and if clinical abnormality then does it every 12 months
- Monitoring in conception, splenectomy and allogenic stem cell transplant are same as TDT

If patient is on hydroxyurea:

- Complete blood counts every 2 weeks for the first 3 months than monthly
- LFT, urea, creatinine every 2 weeks for the first 3 months and then monthly

If patient is planned to give thalidomide:[17]

- CBC with peripheral blood smear to see platelet count
- PT, APTT
- USG doppler study if any swelling and pain in lower limb to see thrombosis
- Anti-HCV Ab

Monitoring of Patients on Thalidomide Therapy[17]

- Menstruation history
- Skin manifestation
- Any swelling and pain of any region

General timelines for monitoring of clinical/lab parameters **(Table 1)** and iron overload **(Table 2)** are summarized below. Details of different iron chelators are summarized in **Table 3.**

TABLE 1: General timeline for clinical and laboratory monitoring.

Initial assessment		Routine test		Clinical test		Laboratory test	Imaging study
Laboratory tests before commencing first blood transfusion		Monthly	3 monthly	6 monthly	Annually	2 yearly	If clinically indicated
CBC with PBS, platelet, morphology of RBC	Other parameters			*For children and adolescent*			
	Molecular study	CBC with PBS	Height	Growth velocity	Bone age	Bone density after 10 years	MRI hypothalamopituitary region
	Blood grouping and ABO Rh typing		Weight	Tanner staging after 11 years	Bone deformity		
	RBC Ag typing extended panel		Serum ferritin, LFT, Urea, cr		FT4, TSH, LH, FSH, GH, calcium, vitamin D3		
	Or		HBsAg, anti HCV Ab, HIV1/2 ab				
	(Kell, c, C, D, E, e)						
				For adults			
Corrected reticulocyte count		CBC with PBS, nRBC, platelet count	Ferritin	Vitamin D3	Audiometry	DXA scan	Lateral spinal X-ray, MRI spine if suspected extramedullary hematopoiesis
			LFT	Serum Ca	Ophthalmoscopy	Echocardiographic TRV	Echocardiographic TRV
			Urea	Uric acid	USG abdomen		HAV, HEV Ab detection
		Any transfusion reaction	Creatinine	FT4, TSH	ECG		Anti HBsAb titre before Hepatitis B vaccination

Continued

Continued

Initial assessment		Routine test		Clinical test		Laboratory test	Imaging study
					For adults		
Serum iron, Ferritin, TIBC			HBsAg		Echocardiography		PT, APTT, fibrinogen, D-dimer
		BP, SpO_2	Anti HCV Ab		Liver fibroscan		CRP, Blood and urine C/S
		Pulse rate	HIV1, 2 Ab		Cardiac MRI T2*		Alpha Feto protein
					Estradiol		MRI of hypothalamo pituitary region
Hb HPLC					Testosterone		DCT
					LH, FSH, OGTT		Creatinine clearance

Clinical assessment of all patients
Every month: Pallor, jaundice, spleen and liver size
Every 3 month: Sitting height, standing height, weight
Every 6 month: Tanner staging

TABLE 2: General timeline for iron overload monitoring.

Routine test		Specific test		
Name of investigation	**Duration interval**	**For cardiac iron overload**	**For liver iron overload**	**For endocrinological iron overload**
Ferritin LFT HCV	3 monthly	ECG	USG abdomen	FT4, TSH, vitamin D3, serum calcium
		2D echocardiography	Liver fibroscan	Serum estradiol, testosterone, LH, FSH Growth hormone
		T2* MRI Echocardiographic TRV	Liver iron concentration by liver biopsy	FBS, PPBS
		All tests to be done every yearly		

TABLE 3: Different iron chelators route of administration, toxicities and monitoring.

Chelators and route of administration	Toxicities	Monitoring recommendation
Deferioxamine (SC or IV)	*Ocular:* • Reduced visual aquity • Decreased field of vision • Abnormal visual evoked potential • Night blindness	Annual eye examination Audiometry annually Serum Zn level annually
	Auditory: • High frequency sensorineural hearing loss • Tinnitus	Sitting and standing height every six months
	Others: • Growth retardation • Zn deficiency • Genu valgum	
Deferasirox (Oral)	*Gastrointestinal:* • Nausea, vomiting, diarrhea, abdominal pain	LFT two weekly initially, then monthly for 6 months and then in every 3 months. Urea, creatinine every three monthly
	Genitourinary: • Increased creatinine • Proteinuria	
Deferiprone (Oral)	• Neutropenia • Agranulocytosis • Arthralgia	CBC with differentials every weekly for 3 months then every monthly

CONCLUSION

Monitoring of thalassemia patients is a vital component of comprehensive care, aiming to minimize complications, prolong survival, and improve quality of life. It requires regular clinical, hematological, biochemical, and radiological assessments with emphasis on detecting and managing iron overload, transfusion-related complications, growth disturbances, endocrinopathies, and organ-specific dysfunction. Careful surveillance also facilitates timely initiation or adjustment of chelation therapy, endocrine interventions, and cardiac or hepatic protection, while addressing special considerations in splenectomized individuals, women planning conception, and patients undergoing hematopoietic stem cell transplantation. Both TDT and NTDT patients benefit from structured follow-up, which remains the cornerstone for reducing morbidity and mortality, tailoring therapy, and ensuring optimal long-term outcomes.

SUMMARY

- *Baseline evaluation*: Includes confirmation of thalassemia type, extended RBC antigen typing (D, C, c, E, e, Kell), baseline CBC, ferritin, liver and renal function tests, viral screening (HBV, HCV, HIV), and anthropometry (height, weight, Tanner staging).
- *Transfusion monitoring*: Maintain pretransfusion hemoglobin between 9.5–10.5 g/dL and post-transfusion < 15 g/dL; use leukoreduced packed RBC; record alloimmunization and transfusion reactions every session.
- *Iron overload assessment*: Serum ferritin every 3 months (chelation if ≥ 1000 ng/mL in TDT or ≥ 800 ng/mL in NTDT); LIC monitoring by MRI T2*, biopsy, or SQUID annually; LIC > 7 mg/g dry weight requires chelation.
- *Cardiac monitoring*: Yearly echocardiography (LVEF, TRV) and MRI T2*; if T2* > 20 ms → monitor biennially; 10–19 ms → annually; <10 ms → high heart-failure risk requiring intensified chelation.
- *Endocrine and growth assessment*: Tanner staging annually (10–17 years), height/weight every 3–6 months, FT4, TSH, GH, LH, FSH, calcium, vitamin D, and parathormone annually to detect hypothyroidism, hypogonadism, and bone disease.
- *Hepatic and renal monitoring*: LFT, urea, and creatinine every 3 months; liver ultrasound biannually; screen for HBV and HCV infection every 3 months; elastography or fibroscan yearly if LIC > 5 mg/g.
- *Bone and metabolic health*: DXA scan of spine and hip annually after 10 years; BMD T-score ≤ -2.5 predicts osteoporosis; wrist/spine X-ray if growth abnormality or deformity.
- *Chelation therapy follow-up*: Monitor ferritin, LFT, urea, creatinine 3-monthly; audiometry and ophthalmic exam annually; CBC weekly for first 3 months on deferiprone, then monthly; evaluate for arthropathy and neutropenia.
- *Special conditions:*
    - *Splenectomized patients*: CBC 3-monthly, TRV yearly, coagulation profile if VTE suspected.
    - *Pregnancy/fertility*: Hormone profile (FT4, TSH, LH, FSH, testosterone, estradiol), USG for ovarian follicle or testicular volume, spouse hemoglobinopathy testing.
- *Non-transfusion-dependent thalassemia (NTDT)*: Monitor ferritin every 3 months, LIC annually, ultrasound abdomen annually, CBC for platelet/nRBC count, DXA every 1–2 years, and screen for pulmonary hypertension and extramedullary hematopoiesis by TRV and MRI as indicated.
- *HSCT candidates*: HLA typing (<17 years), ferritin, LFT, urea, creatinine every 3 months; iron control and infection screening prior to conditioning; post-transplant monitoring as per hematopoietic cell transplant protocols.

REFERENCES

1. Taher AT, Musallam KM, Cappellini MD. beta-Thalassemias. N Engl J Med. 2021;384(8):727-43.
2. Kattamis A, Kwiatkowski JL, Aydinok Y. Thalassaemia. Lancet. 2022;399(10343):2310-24.
3. Cazzola M, De Stefano P, Ponchio L, et al. Relationship between transfusion regimen and suppression of erythropoiesis in beta-thalassaemia major. Br J Haematol. 1995;89(3):473-8.
4. Danjou F, Francavilla M, Anni F, et al. A genetic score for the prediction of beta-thalassemia severity. Haematologica. 2015;100(4):452-7.
5. Cazzola M, Borgna-Pignatti C, Locatelli F, et al. A moderate transfusion regimen may reduce iron loading in beta-thalassemia major without producing excessive expansion of erythropoiesis. Transfusion. 1997;37(2):135-40.
6. Saiviroonporn P, Viprakasit V, Sanpakit K, et al. Intersite validations of the pixel-wise method for liver R2* analysis in transfusion-dependent thalassemia patients: a more accessible and affordable diagnostic technology. Hematol Oncol Stem Cell Ther. 2012;5(2):91-5.
7. Kirk P, He T, Anderson LJ, et al. International reproducibility of single breathhold T2* MR for cardiac and liver iron assessment among five thalassemia centers. J Magn Reson Imaging. 2010;32(2):315-9.
8. Adamkiewicz TV, Abboud MR, Paley C, et al. Serum ferritin level changes in children with sickle cell disease on chronic blood transfusion are nonlinear and are associated with iron load and liver injury. Blood. 2009;114(21):4632-8.
9. Anderson LJ, Westwood MA, Holden S, et al. Myocardial iron clearance during reversal of siderotic cardiomyopathy with intravenous desferrioxamine: a prospective study using T2* cardiovascular magnetic resonance. British Journal of Haematology. 2004;127(3):348-55.
10. Angelucci E, Brittenham GM, McLaren CE, et al. Hepatic iron concentration and total body iron stores in thalassemia major. N Engl J Med. 2000;343(5):327-31.
11. St Pierre TG, Clark PR, Chua-anusorn W, et al. Noninvasive measurement and imaging of liver iron concentrations using proton magnetic resonance. Blood. 2005;105(2):855-61.
12. Behzadifar M, Gorji HA, Bragazzi NL. The prevalence of hepatitis C virus infection in thalassemia patients in Iran from 2000 to 2017: a systematic review and meta-analysis. Arch Virol. 2018;163(5):1131-40.
13. Ayidinok Y, Kattamis A, Cappellini MD, et al. Deferasirox-deferoxamine combination therapy reduces cardiac iron with rapid liver iron removal after 24 months in patients with severe transfusional iron overload (HYPERION). Haematologica. 2014;99:229.
14. Bajoria R, Chatterjee R. Current perspectives of fertility and pregnancy in thalassemia. Hemoglobin. 2009;33 Suppl 1:S131-5.
15. Casale M, Cinque P, Ricchi P, et al. Effect of splenectomy on iron balance in patients with β-thalassemia major: a long-term follow-up. European Journal of Haematology. 2013;91(1): 69-73.
16. Anurathapan U, Hongeng S, Pakakasama S, et al. Hematopoietic Stem Cell Transplantation for Severe Thalassemia Patients from Haploidentical Donors Using a Novel Conditioning Regimen. Biol Blood Marrow Transplant. 2020;26(6): 1106-12.
17. Lu Y, Wei Z, Yang G, et al. Investigating the efficacy and safety of thalidomide for treating patients with s-thalassemia: A meta-analysis. Front. Pharmacol. 2022;12:814302.

11 CHAPTER

Fetal Hemoglobin Induction in Beta-thalassemia

AK Tripathi, Shailendra Prasad Verma

INTRODUCTION

Beta-thalassemia is a group of inherited blood disorders caused by mutations in the *HBB* gene, resulting in the reduced synthesis of beta-globin chains. The severity of the disease varies based on the type and number of mutations. Patients with beta-thalassemia experience hemolytic anemia, splenomegaly, and iron overload due to frequent blood transfusions.[1,2] Currently, the only curative treatment for beta-thalassemia is allogeneic hematopoietic stem cell transplantation (HSCT).[3] However, this procedure is associated with significant risks and limited availability of suitable donors. Hence, alternative therapeutic strategies are required to manage the condition effectively.

FETAL HEMOGLOBIN AND ITS ROLE IN BETA-THALASSEMIA

Fetal hemoglobin (HbF) is the primary oxygen-carrying hemoglobin during fetal life, composed of two alpha-globin and two gamma-globin chains ($\alpha2\gamma2$). After birth, gamma-globin expression is repressed, and the production of adult hemoglobin (HbA, $\alpha2\beta2$) takes over.[4] In patients with beta-thalassemia, the increased expression of HbF can ameliorate the clinical manifestations by partially compensating for the reduced production of functional beta-globin chains.[3,4] This observation has triggered research efforts to understand the regulatory mechanisms governing HbF expression and identify strategies to enhance its production.[5] The **Figure 1** below shows the switch of hemoglobin during embryonic life and after birth.

Genetic Basis of Fetal Hemoglobin Induction

The regulation of HbF expression is complex and involves multiple genetic loci and regulatory elements. Genome-wide association studies (GWAS) have identified several genetic variants associated with elevated HbF levels in both thalassemia and nonthalassemia populations. Among the key regulators of HbF expression are the *BCL11A* and *MYB* genes, as well as the HBS1L-MYB intergenic region.[5,6] These genes and regions serve as potential targets for therapeutic intervention to induce HbF in beta-thalassemia.

Fetal hemoglobin induction is a complex process regulated by genetic factors, epigenetic modifications, and various signaling pathways. Understanding the genetic basis of fetal hemoglobin induction is crucial for developing targeted therapeutic approaches to treat hemoglobin disorders like beta-

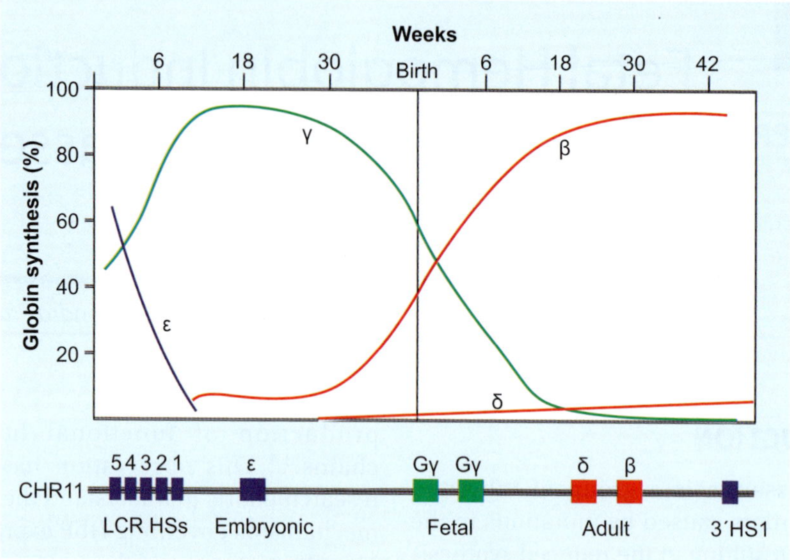

FIG. 1: The switch of Hemoglobin during embryonic life and after birth.

thalassemia and sickle cell disease. Here, we explore the key genetic components involved in fetal hemoglobin regulation:

- *Gamma-globin gene cluster*: The gamma-globin gene cluster, located on chromosome 11 in humans, is responsible for encoding the globin chains of fetal hemoglobin. This cluster includes two main genes: The embryonic ε-globin gene (HBG1) and the fetal γ-globin gene (HBG2). During fetal development, these genes are actively transcribed to produce HbF.
- *Silencing of gamma-globin genes*: After birth, there is a switch from HbF to adult hemoglobin (HbA), primarily composed of alpha and beta globin chains. This switch is tightly regulated, and the gamma-globin genes are usually silenced or suppressed in adults. The mechanisms responsible for this silencing involve various transcription factors and regulatory elements.
- *Repressors of gamma-globin genes*: One of the key repressors of fetal hemoglobin production is BCL11A (B-cell lymphoma/leukemia 11A). BCL11A acts as a transcriptional repressor that binds to specific DNA sequences in the promoters of gamma-globin genes, inhibiting their expression. Genetic variations in the *BCL11A* gene have been associated with altered HbF levels in individuals with hemoglobin disorders.
- *Genetic modifiers*: Several genetic modifiers have been identified that influence the levels of fetal hemoglobin in individuals with hemoglobin disorders. For example, single nucleotide polymorphisms (SNPs) in the HBS1L-MYB intergenic region on chromosome 6 have been found to be associated with HbF levels.
- *Epigenetic modifications*: Epigenetic changes, such as DNA methylation and histone modifications, play a critical role in regulating fetal hemoglobin expression. DNA methylation, in particular, is involved in silencing the gamma-globin genes in adult red blood cells. Epigenetic modifiers,

such as DNA methyl transferase inhibitors and histone deacetylase inhibitors, have been explored as potential therapeutic agents to induce HbF expression.

- *Transcription factors and enhancers*: Several transcription factors and enhancer elements are involved in regulating the expression of gamma-globin genes. For example, the transcription factors GATA-1 and KLF1 are essential for the proper expression of fetal hemoglobin during development.
- *Chromatin remodeling*: The chromatin structure of the gamma-globin genes undergoes dynamic changes during development, influencing their accessibility to transcription factors and RNA polymerase. Chromatin remodeling complexes and regulatory elements modulate this process and impact HbF induction.
- *Long non-coding RNAs (lncRNAs)*: Long non-coding RNAs are emerging as important regulators of gene expression, including the gamma-globin genes. Certain lncRNAs have been found to interact with transcription factors and chromatin remodeling complexes to influence fetal hemoglobin expression.

Advances in genetic and epigenetic research have provided valuable insights into the mechanisms governing fetal hemoglobin expression. Targeting specific regulators, such as BCL11A, through gene-editing techniques and pharmacological interventions, shows promise as potential therapeutic strategies. Continued research in this area holds the potential to revolutionize the treatment of hemoglobin disorders and improve the quality of life for affected individuals.

Primary and Secondary Modifiers[7]

- *Primary modifiers*: These modifiers directly affect the HbF levels. β globin gene mutations and presence of α-thalassemia are considered to be primary modifiers of HbF induction.
- *Secondary modifiers*: It can influence the clinical presentation of the disease by impacting other factors that affect the imbalance of globin chains. Genetic variants associated with increased HbF levels such as BCL11A, HBS1L-MIB, KLF1 variations and HBG2 polymorphisms are considered as secondary modifiers of HbF induction.

PHARMACOLOGICAL APPROACHES TO FETAL HEMOGLOBIN INDUCTION

Various pharmacological agents have been investigated for their potential to induce fetal hemoglobin production. Some of the commonly studied agents include.

Hydroxyurea

Hydroxyurea is one of the most well-known fetal hemoglobin inducers and has been used in the treatment of beta-thalassemia and sickle cell disease. Hydroxyurea therapy exerts a 2- to 9-fold increase in γ-mRNA expression in β-thalassemia patients. It acts by increasing the production of nitric oxide, which in turn activates guanylate cyclase, leading to increased levels of cGMP and gamma-globin gene expression. Toxicity of hydroxyurea is mainly myelosuppression and it is reversible upon dose reduction or cessation. Other side effects are nail changes, hyperpigmentation, cutaneous vasculitis/ulcers, nausea, vomiting and anorexia.

In beta-thalassemia it can lead to increased HbF levels, reduced transfusion dependency, and decreased complications like skeletal deformities. Hydroxyurea has modest responses in β thalassemia major patients at doses 10–15 mg/kg body weight. Studies by Bradai et al. and Koren et al. showed that around 45 and 90% patients showed good response with a rise of 1.5 g/dL and Hb mean of 8.2 ± 0.7 g/dL respectively in these studies. In thalassemia intermedia the responses are even better because α/β globin imbalance is lesser. A study by Karimi M et al. including 163 patients of thalassemia intermedia showed 149/163 (91.4%) response to HU. The mean Hb level was 9.5 g/dL. All patients were treated with HU 8–12 mg/kg/day orally once a day.[8,9]

Thalidomide

Thalidomide is an immunomodulatory drug which can induce HbF by modulating *GATA1* and *KLF* gene expression. It can reduce the transfusion needs in thalassemia patients. A very recent study by Rahman et al. including 164 TDT patients showed that hemoglobin level in the thalidomide group significantly increased from 6.12 ± 0.65 to 8.36 ± 2.04 g/dL ($p < 0.001$). Among thalidomide-treated patients, 34.7% were excellent responders (ER), 25% good responders (GR), 13.9% partial responders (PR), and 26.4% nonresponders (NR). Usual proposed doses of thalidomide is 50–100 mg/day.[10]

Butyrate Derivatives

Compounds such as arginine butyrate or sodium phenylbutyrate have been shown to enhance fetal hemoglobin production by promoting histone acetylation, which leads to changes in chromatin structure and increased gamma-globin gene transcription.

Decitabine

Decitabine is a cytosine analogue and a DNA methyltransferase inhibitor that has demonstrated the ability to reactivate fetal hemoglobin expression by reducing DNA methylation in the gamma-globin gene promoters. Low dose decitabine 0.2 mg/kg body weight twice per week for 12 weeks is also effective.

Pomalidomide

This immunomodulatory drug has shown promise in inducing fetal hemoglobin production by an as-yet-unknown mechanism.

Short-chain Fatty Acids

Compounds like valproic acid and phenylbutyrate have shown potential as fetal hemoglobin inducers by acting on histone deacetylases.

BCL11A Inhibitors

BCL11A is a key repressor of fetal hemoglobin production in adults. Inhibition of BCL11A has shown promise in preclinical studies as a potential strategy for HbF induction in beta-thalassemia. Various small molecule inhibitors and gene-editing techniques (e.g., CRISPR-Cas9) were being investigated to target BCL11A and reactivate fetal hemoglobin expression.[11]

HDAC Inhibitors

Histone deacetylase (HDAC) inhibitors have been studied for their potential to induce fetal hemoglobin expression. By blocking HDAC enzymes, these agents promote histone acetylation, leading to increased gamma-globin gene transcription.

Mithramycin

Mithramycin is an antibiotic that has shown promising results in preclinical studies for fetal hemoglobin induction in beta-thalassemia. It works by binding to the gamma-globin promoter region and promoting gamma-globin gene expression.

BET Protein Inhibitors

Bromodomain and extraterminal (BET) protein inhibitors have been investigated for their ability to modulate gamma-globin gene expression. These inhibitors target BET proteins that regulate gene transcription and have shown potential in preclinical studies.

NEWER APPROACHES

Gene therapy and genome editing for HbF induction: Refer to chapter on Recent Advances (Chapter 18).

CHALLENGES AND FUTURE DIRECTIONS

- Despite the significant progress made in fetal hemoglobin induction for beta-thalassemia, several challenges remain to be addressed.
- The heterogeneity of thalassemia mutations, the variable responses to HbF-inducing agents, and the potential off-target effects of gene editing are some of the hurdles that need to be overcome.
- Additionally, large-scale clinical trials are necessary to establish the safety and efficacy of these therapies.

CONCLUSION

Fetal hemoglobin induction in beta-thalassemia holds promise as a therapeutic approach to alleviate the burden of this inherited blood disorder. Advances in understanding the genetic basis of HbF regulation and the development of pharmacological and gene-based strategies have provided hope for more effective treatments and even cures. Continued research and clinical trials will be crucial to realizing the full potential of these therapeutic interventions, ultimately improving the quality of life for individuals living with beta-thalassemia.

SUMMARY

1. HbF induction is one of the promising strategy to decreased transfusion requirements and improve clinical outcomes in patients with thalassemia.
2. Clinical improvement is expected to be better in β-thalassemia intermedia patients compared to TDT.
3. Hydroxyurea has shown clinical efficacy in thalassemia patients and should be tried in doses of 10–15 mg/kg with close monitoring of side effects.
4. Thalidomide is another promising immunomodulatory agent used in doses of 50–100 mg/day.
5. More studies and a promising targeted approach is needed to induce HbF in thalassemia patients.

REFERENCES

1. Weatherall DJ, Clegg JB. The Thalassemia Syndromes, 4th edition. Philadelphia: Blackwell Science, 2001.
2. Orkin SH, Nathan DG, Ginsburg D, et al. Nathan and Oski's Hematology and Oncology of Infancy and Childhood, 8th edition. Philadelphia: Saunders; 2015.
3. Galanello R, Origa R. Beta-thalassemia. Orphanet J Rare Dis. 2010;5:11.
4. Sankaran VG, Orkin SH. The switch from fetal to adult hemoglobin. Cold Spring Harb Perspect Med. 2013;3(1):a011643.
5. Bauer DE, Kamran SC, Orkin SH, et al. Advances in the understanding of g-globin gene regulation and implications for gene therapy for beta-globin disorders. Exp Hematol. 2018;66:16-31.
6. Mabaera R, West RJ, Conine SJ, et al. A cell stress signaling model of fetal hemoglobin induction: what doesn't kill red blood cells may make them stronger. Exp Hematol. 2008;36(9):1057-72.
7. Thein SL. Genetic modifiers of beta-thalassemia. Haematologica. 2005;90(5):649-60.
8. Bradai M, Abad MT, Pissard S, et al. Hydroxyurea can eliminate transfusion requirements in

children with severe beta-thalassemia. Blood. 2003;102(4):1529-30.
9. Karimi M, Darzi H, Yavarian M. Hematologic and clinical responses of thalassemia intermedia patients to hydroxyurea during 6 years of therapy in Iran. J Pediatr Hematol Oncol. 2005;27(7):380-5.
10. Rahman I U, Khan MTM, Ali Z, et al. Thalidomide confers therapeutic benefit in beta thalassemia patients by enhancing hemoglobin and hematopoietic gene expression: A non-randomized clinical trial. Blood Cells Mol Dis. 2025;113-114:102936.
11. Mettananda S, Fisher CA, Hay D, et al. Editing an α-globin enhancer in primary human hematopoietic stem cells as a treatment for β-thalassemia. Nat Commun. 2017;8(1):424.

12

CHAPTER

Thalassemia—Complications and Management

Jina Bhattacharyya, Damodar Das, Sweta Das

INTRODUCTION

Thalassemia, both transfusion-dependent thalassemia (TDT) and nontransfusion-dependent thalassemia (NTDT) can cause different types of complications involving different organ systems. Adequate management of these complications require a multidisciplinary approach.

- *Iron overload*: Refer to chapter on Iron Overload
- *Endocrine complications*: Refer to chapter on Endocrine Complications
- *Skeletal Complications*: Refer to chapter on Endocrine complications and Imaging in Thalassemia
- *Cardiac complications*: Refer to chapter on Cardiac Evaluation
- *Hepatic complications*: Refer to chapter on Iron Overload
- *Others*: Described below

THROMBOEMBOLIC COMPLICATIONS IN PATIENTS WITH THALASSEMIA

Beta-thalassemia patients are in a hyper-coagulable state and thromboembolic events (TEE) are unique features of the disease. These can occur both in TDT and NTDT patients with higher incidence reported in the latter.[1] In a study involving 8,860 patients, the prevalence has been reported as 1.65% in thalassemia major (TM) and 4.38% in thalassemia minor (TI) patients.[2] This study has identified the following, as risk factors for having TEE:

- Splenectomy
- Family history of thrombosis
- Age >20 years
- TI patients (NTDT)

These were further confirmed by subsequent studies;[3-5] In addition to these, Hb > 9 g/dL/transfusion naivety were recognized as risk factors for TEE. In a 10-year follow up study of splenectomized patients (n = 79), 29% patients had TEE confirming further, that post splenectomized patients are at risk of TEE.

Thus thrombotic complications are four-fold higher in NTDT than in TDT patients; the risk increases with age; it is seen in 28.2% in NTDT patients above the age of 35 years as compared to those between 18–35 years (14.9%) and 4.1% in patients younger than 18 years of age.[2] Incidence of overt strokes is relatively low (5%) and it occurs more frequently in TM than TI (28% vs. 9%); but it has been shown by MRI that as many as 37.5% TI have brain damage on MRI. However silent strokes have been reported in as high as 60% of splenectomized adults (mean age, 32 years) with NTDT.[6] **Figure 1** shows the TEE in TM versus TI.

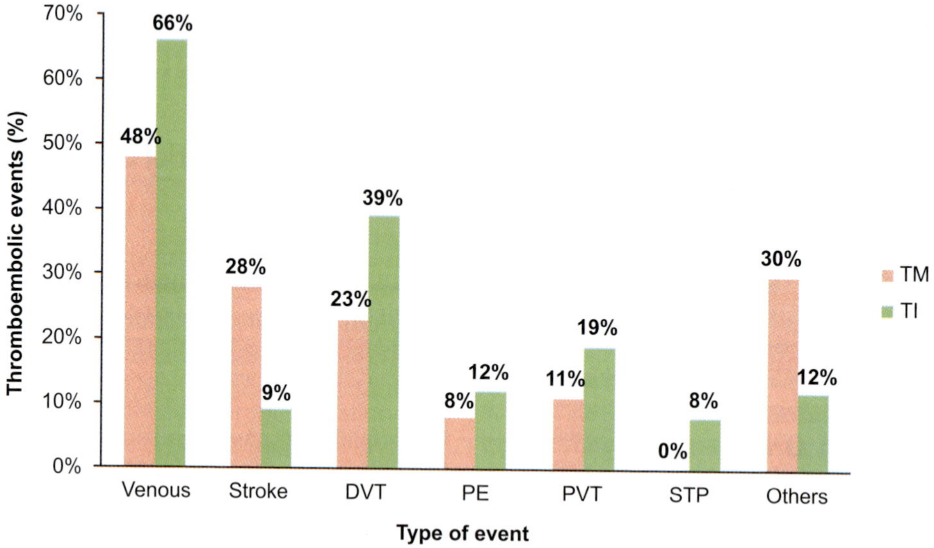

FIG. 1: Incidence of thromboembolic events in TM and TI patients. (TM: thalassemia major; TI: thalassemia intermedia)

WHAT IS PATHOPHYSIOLOGY?

Multiple factors are involved in the pathogenesis of TEE in patients with thalassemia.[7] Disease-specific features and thrombotic features are combined to result in TEE in these patients.

Changes in RBCs

Due to imbalance in alpha and beta chains, the RBCs of thalassemia patients form hemichromes from oxidated hemoglobin; as a result heme disintegrates to release non transferrin bound Iron (NTBI) and reactive oxygen species (ROS); these result in alteration of RBC membranes which provide a procoagulant surface for the activation of the coagulation cascade.

Hemolysis of the RBCs also act as a triggering factor; release of hemoglobin and heme stimulates endothelial activation and tissue factor expression; there is also a reduction of nitric oxide (NO) which in turn leads to platelet activation and vasoconstriction.

Changes in Platelets

There is a state of chronic activation of platelets in patients with thalassemia; this has been shown by findings of increased expression of markers of platelet activation and aggregation (P-selectin and CD63).

Changes in the Endothelium

There is endothelial activation and injury in patients with thalassemia as evidenced by increased levels of endothelial adhesion molecules, e.g., E-selectin (ELAM-1), intercellular adhesion molecule 1 (ICAM-1), vascular cell adhesion molecule (VCAM-1) and von Willebrand Factor (VWF); these activated endothelial cells interact with white blood cells (WBC). These cellular interactions between WBCs, RBCs, platelets, endothelial cells, procoagulant cytokines and vasoconstriction mediated by dysregulated NO result in TEE in thalassemic patients.

Presence of Microparticles

Microparticles (MP) which have procoagulant properties are identified in thalassemia patients; these MPs are derived from the hemolyzed RBCs, endothelial cells, WBCs and activated platelets

Splenectomy

Splenectomy has been identified as the risk factor for causing TEE. Thrombocytosis and platelet hyperactivity following splenectomy, increased number of abnormal circulating RBCs due to loss of splenic clearance and externalized negatively charged phospholipids are the causes for patients being at risk of TEE.

Iron Overload, ROS, and Complement

Iron overload can lead to formation of ROS which are responsible for oxidative tissue damage, vascular injury and platelet activation. Complement also has been implicated in the causation of TEE; complement activation occurs due to free heme.

Thrombophilia

Associated thrombophilic state, either congenital or acquired, put patients with thalassemia at risk of TEE. Decreased levels of protein C, protein S, and antithrombin III, as well as the presence of anti-phospholipid antibodies, have been associated with TEE in these patients.

Other Factors

Underlying disorders like hepatic dysfunction, cardiac dysfunction, and endocrine disorders put the patients of thalassemia at risk of developing TEE.

HOW DO WE MANAGE AN ACUTE EPISODE?

The approach to all acute episodes of thrombosis are similar to those for nonthalassemic patients. Anticoagulants and antiplatelets remain the cornerstone of management of acute events.

Guidelines are there for both acute episodes and for thromboprophylaxis. **Figure 2** shows the general recommendations of treating patients with TEE.

Choices of anticoagulants are:
- *Antiplatelets*: Low-dose ecosprin
- Low molecular weight heparin or unfractionated heparin
- *Coumarin derivatives*: Warfarin or acitrom

Direct acting oral anticoagulants (DOAC) **(Table 1)**:
- *Direct Xa inhibitor*: Rivaroxaban, apixaban, and edoxaban
- *Direct thrombin inhibitor*: Dabigatran

With the introduction of DOAC [TOAC (targeted oral anticoagulant)], more and more VTEs are being treated with these, except in certain situations like prosthetic valves where DOACs are contraindicated. Direct thrombin inhibitors are available as capsules as well as oral solutions for use in pediatrics. DOACs are approved for pediatric use except below 3 months of age. The dose is calculated based on body weight of the child.

Half-lives of Different DOACs (Table 2)

All are excreted through the renal route.

Antidote for the DOACs are: For direct IIa inhibitor, it is idarucizumab and for direct Xa inhibitors, it is andexanet-α.

Dose interruption is done for any procedure or surgery; these are to be stopped 24 hours prior to the procedure and restarted 12 hours post procedure.

DOACs are presently not indicated in children with mechanical valves, triple-positive APLA syndrome, severe liver or kidney diseases, those with limited GI absorption, or those on concomitant medications that are inducers and inhibitors of CYP3A4 and P-gp.

Acute period (first 5–21 days)	Long-term period (3–6 months)	Extended period (beyond long-term period)
UFH/LMWH lead-in (first 5–10 days)	Warfarin: Within therapeutic target INR level	If required
UFH/LMWH lead-in (first 5–10 days)	LMWH (in cases of cancer-associated thrombosis): Therapeutic dose	If required
UFH/LMWH lead-in (first 5 days)	Edoxaban: 60 mg q.d. (30 mg/day if body weight <60 kg or CrCl 30–50 min/mL)	If required
UFH/LMWH lead-in (first 5 days)	Dabigatran: 150 mg b.i.d.	If required
Rivaroxaban 15 mg b.i.d. (first 21 days)	20 mg q.d. instead of b.i.d.	If required: 10 mg q.d.
Apixaban: 10 mg b.i.d. (first 7 days)	Apixaban: 5 mg b.i.d.	If required: 2.5 mg b.i.d.

FIG. 2: Treatment recommendation of VEE.

TABLE 1: Mechanism of action of direct oral anticoagulants (DOACs).

Dabigatran etexilate	Rivaroxaban	Apixaban	Edoxaban
Direct IIa inhibitor; inhibits clot-bound and free thrombin	Direct Xa inhibitor; inhibits clot-bound and free Xa	Direct Xa inhibitor; inhibits clot-bound and free Xa	Direct Xa inhibitor; inhibits clot-bound and free Xa

TABLE 2: Half-life of direct oral anticoagulants (DOACs).

Debgatran	Rivaroxaban	Apixaban	Edoxaban
12–17 h	5–9 h	8–12 h	10–14 hours

Thromboprophylaxis

It has been shown that patients treated with antiplatelets have a lower risk of recurrence compared to those who did not receive antiplatelets.[8]

It is recommended to give thromboprophylaxis to patients who are at risk. Patients are risk stratified based on presence of any thalassemia related or non-thalassemia related risk factors; like NTDT patients, splenectomized patients, patients with Hb of less than 9 g/dL, high NRBCs, and high platelet counts, older age, pregnancy, malignancy, history of thrombosis in the past or in the family, major surgery or immobilization.

Choices of Drugs for Prophylaxis

Based on the nature of the risk factor the particular thromboprophylactic drug is selected; choices of drug also depend on availability, cost and patients' choice.

In patients who have been splenectomized and have thrombocytosis, antiplatelet drug is the choice; low dose aspirin (75 mg) is recommended for this group of patients. Aspirin is not recommended for thalassemia patients with cardiovascular disorders due to aspirin resistance.[9] For patients with atrial fibrillation (AF) in thalassemics, both LMWH or UFH can be used but warfarin is used most commonly in this group of patients.[10]

Duration Anticoagulants

Depending upon the risk factors, the duration of thromboprophylaxis can be decided, e.g., if a patient of NTDT is started on thromboprophylaxis during pregnancy, the same can be stopped 6 weeks postpartum as per the thromboprophylaxis guideline for the general population.

Other Prophylactic Measures for VEE Prevention

As transfusion naivety has been identified as a risk factor for VEE, therapeutic strategy may be changed in NTDT patients by giving regular transfusion but this decision has to be taken by assessing the benefit of it to outweigh the risk of regular transfusion. Likewise splenectomy is advised only when there is absolute indication, e.g., hypersplenism and symptomatic splenomegaly.

MONITORING FOR VEE

There is no monitoring guideline; however a clinical scoring system has been introduced by Taher et al.[11] for risk stratification and treatment decision. **Table 3** shows the thalassemia related thrombosis risk scoring system (TRT-RSS)

TABLE 3: TRT-RSS.

Risk factor at time of assessment	Score	Risk category
Age >35	2.5	TRT-RSS risk min = 0
Hb level >9 g/dL	2.5	TRT-RSS max = 17
S Ferritin level >1000 mcg/L	2.0	
Not regularly transfused	3.5	LR <9.5
Splenectomized	6.5	IR 9.5-13.5
		HR >13.5

Figure 1 shows VEE in TM versus TI.

Treatment recommendations for VEE are summarized in **Figure 2**.

Recommendations

- All patients with thalassemia should be risk stratified for VEE risk.
- Thromboprophylaxis is recommended for all those who are at risk.
- Acute cases are treated as per existing guideline for general population with either LMWH and warfarin or DOAC.
- Low-dose aspirin is to be given to splenectomized patients with thrombocytosis.
- Aspirin is avoided in thalassemia patients with cardiovascular disorders.

LEG ULCER

Chronic leg ulcers are seen in patients with inherited hemoglobin disorders. There is dearth of published data about leg ulcer in thalassemia patients; few available data shows that the leg ulcers are more commonly seen in patients with NTDT than in TDT.[12-14]

Amongst the NTDT patients, leg ulcers has been reported to be more common in patients with HbE beta-thalassemia, with a reported prevalence of 22% in a single center study.[15]

What are the Risk Factors?

One of the primary risk factors identified in different studies is severe untreated or undertreated chronic anemia.[15] The risk increases with advancing age. Ineffective erythropoiesis, splenectomy and hypercoagulable state are also identified as risk factors for ulcer development.[16-20] Iron overload is another risk factor for development of leg ulcer in NTDT patients.[21] Elevated level of fetal Hb (HbF) has also been shown to aggravate tissue hypoxia leading to chronic leg ulcer.

Ongoing red cell hemolysis leads to consumption of nitric oxide and impaired endothelial function which can also lead to formation of leg ulcers.

Exposure of the leg ulcer in tropical countries and trauma can be inciting factors for the development of leg ulcer.

Presence of comorbidities like diabetes mellitus puts the patients at risk of leg ulcer development.

How to Treat Leg Ulcer?

Leg ulcers are indolent and painful; they are slow to heal and have a significant impact on the quality of life of the patients. Approach to treatment can be divided into local care and systemic treatment.

A multidisciplinary team should include a dermatologist, plastic surgeon, nutritionists and a hematologist.

Local Care

- *Regular dressing of ulcer*: Cleansing, debridement of dead tissue, and antiseptic dressing are to be done regularly.
- Compression bandage can be used to improve circulation

Systemic Care

- Blood transfusion, hydroxycarbamide (hydroxyurea), pentoxifylline can help in healing of leg ulcers.
- Vasodilators like diazepam (adenosine reuptake inhibitor) have been shown to be beneficial in patients with E beta-thalassemia.[21]
- Patients can be treated with skin grafting, negative pressure wound therapy may be needed in refractory cases.
- Some patients can be benefitted by platelet derived wound healing factors and granulocyte macrophage colony stimulating factors. Sodium nitrite solution has been shown to be beneficial in patients with refractory leg ulcers.[22]
- Luspatercept is a drug, which is used to treat anemia that has shown healing of leg ulcer.[23]

Preventive Strategies

- *Avoidance of trauma*: Appropriate foot wear, proper hygiene and avoiding skin breakdown
- *Regular leg care*: Prompt care of any wound
- Elevation of legs, avoiding prolonged standing would avoid venous insufficiency

Recommendation for Leg Ulcer

- NTDT patients are at higher risk of developing leg ulcers.
- Advancing age, splenectomy, under-transfusion, patients with Hb < 10 g/dL, iron overload and patients with low fetal hemoglobin are risk factors for development of leg ulcers.
- All high-risk patients should be monitored closely
- The skin of the patient with high risk should be monitored routinely.
- A team of doctors including a dermatologist and a plastic surgeon should be collaborating in treating leg ulcers.
- Simple measures like raising the foot end while sleeping would help
- Topical application of antibiotics and sodium nitrite

- In patients with persistent leg ulcers, blood transfusion, hydroxyurea and luspatercept are the choices of treatment.

CHOLELITHIASIS/GALLSTONE DISEASE IN THALASSEMIA

Patients with thalassemia are at increased risk of developing gallstones. Cholelithiasis is defined by radiological evidence of presence of gallstones;[24] the reported incidence of gallstones in patients with thalassemia is 10-57% of TM patients.[24-26]

Why do Thalassemia Patients get Gallstones?

Pathogenesis of gallstones in thalassemia patients is multifactorial. The primary factor is the chronic hemolysis in patients with thalassemia;[27] this leads to increased bilirubin production which gets precipitated as calcium bilirubinate in the bile leading to formation of pigment gallstones.

Iron deposition in the gallbladder also leads to formation of gallstones.[28] Iron Overload due to disease and frequent blood transfusions lead to iron overload, which may further affect bile metabolism and increase gallstone formation risk.

Ineffective erythropoiesis or red blood cell production in the bone marrow is an important contributing factor leading to higher bilirubin levels and gallstone formation.[29]

Studies suggest that bile in thalassemia patients may have altered properties, such as decreased contractility of the gallbladder, leading to slower bile flow and potentially promoting stone formation.[30]

Other factors significantly related to cholelithiasis are older age, magnitude of transfusion and splenectomy.[25,31]

Formation of gallstones itself leads to complications like cholecystitis, choledocholithiasis and acute pancreatitis. Cholecystitis occurs as a result of inflammation of the gallbladder causing fever, pain, nausea and vomiting. Choledocholithiasis results from migration of gallstones into the common bile duct, causing obstruction and infection of the bile duct (cholangitis). Acute Pancreatitis occurs when blocked bile ducts cause inflammation of the pancreas.

Management of Gallstones in Thalassemia

Monitoring for gallstone disease is an important component of management. Regular ultrasound screenings, once in 6 months is recommended to detect gallstones early more so in patients with thalassemia intermedia.

Cholecystectomy is recommended for all symptomatic patients irrespective of age to prevent complications. Laparoscopic surgery is recommended unless otherwise indicated.

Emergency surgery should be avoided as far as possible. Therefore, it is recommended to plan elective surgery even in asymptomatic patients with specified indications to avoid emergency surgery. Due to the increased risk of complications associated with acute cholecystitis in thalassemia patients, some studies advocate for elective cholecystectomy even in asymptomatic cases, especially in children and individuals with other comorbidities.

If the patient is planned for splenectomy, and has gallstones, cholecystectomy is recommended in the same sitting, even though the patient is asymptomatic.

Some patients may need endoscopic retrograde cholangiopancreatography (ERCP) to remove stones from the bile duct before or during cholecystectomy.

It's important to note that the decision regarding the timing of surgery (elective vs. symptomatic) should be made in consultation with a multidisciplinary team, considering the individual patient's condition, severity of thalassemia, and the presence of other co-morbidities. It is of utmost significance that patients with thalassemia undergoing cholecystectomy require special care in terms of transfusion, wound care and close monitoring and the team of doctors must work together to minimize complication.

CONCLUSION

Thalassemia can lead to a range of complications impacting various organ systems, including hematologic, skeletal, cardiac, hepatic, endocrine, immune systems. Besides these, complications like VTE, cholelithiasis and leg ulcers contribute to the HR-QOL of thalassemia patients. Knowledge and identification of these complications, taking preventive measures and timely and adequate treatment can give a good QOL to patients with thalassemia.

SUMMARY

- *Multisystem impact*: Thalassemia (both TDT and NTDT) causes complications involving hematologic, cardiovascular, hepatic, skeletal, and endocrine systems, mainly due to ineffective erythropoiesis, chronic hemolysis, and iron overload.
- *Thromboembolic events (TEE)*: NTDT patients show higher risk (4.38%) than TDT (1.65%); contributing factors include splenectomy, age >20 years, transfusion naivety, high Hb >9 g/dL, and platelet activation.
- *Pathophysiology of thrombosis*: Hemichrome formation, oxidative injury, RBC and platelet activation, endothelial dysfunction, microparticles, complement activation, and thrombophilia jointly promote a prothrombotic state.
- *Acute thrombosis management*: Use low-molecular-weight heparin, warfarin, or direct oral anticoagulants (dabigatran, rivaroxaban, apixaban, edoxaban); DOACs require renal monitoring and antidotes (idarucizumab for IIa, andexanet-α for Xa inhibitors).
- *Thromboprophylaxis*: High-risk patients (splenectomized, NTDT, high platelets, low Hb, pregnancy, history of VTE) should receive low-dose aspirin (75 mg) or warfarin where indicated; aspirin avoided in cardiovascular comorbidities.
- *Leg ulcers*: More common in NTDT and E-β thalassemia (≈22% prevalence); risk factors include chronic anemia, splenectomy, iron overload, hemolysis, and advancing age.
  Management: Local wound care, compression therapy, hydroxyurea, pentoxifylline, vasodilators, and luspatercept; skin grafts or sodium nitrite for refractory cases.
- *Gallstone disease*: Occurs in 10–57% of thalassemia patients; primarily from chronic hemolysis, bilirubin supersaturation, and iron overload; aggravated by age, splenectomy, and gallbladder dysmotility.
- *Cholelithiasis management*: Six-monthly ultrasound screening recommended; symptomatic or high-risk cases need laparoscopic cholecystectomy; consider concurrent surgery during splenectomy.

REFERENCES

1. Borgna-Pignatti C, Rugolotto S, DeStefano P, et al. Survival and complications in patients with thalassemia major treated with transfusion and deferoxamine. Haematologica. 2004;89(10):1187-93.
2. Taher A, Isma'eel H, Mehio G, et al. Prevalence of thromboembolic events among 8,860 patients with thalassaemia major and intermedia in the Mediterranean area and Iran: Thromb. Haemostasis. 2006;96(4):488-91.

3. Taher AT, Musallam K, Karimi M, et al. Overview on practices in thalassemia intermedia management aiming for lowering complication rates across a region of endemicity: the OPTIMAL CARE study. Blood. 2010;115(10):1886-92.
4. Cappellini MD, Robbiolo L, Bottasso BM, et al. Mannucci Venous thromboembolism and hypercoagulability in splenectomized patients with thalassaemia intermedia. Br. J. Haematol. 2000;111(2):467-73.
5. Taher AT, Musallam KM, Karimi M, et al. Splenectomy and thrombosis: the case of thalassemia intermedia. J Thromb Haemostasis. 2010;8:2152-8.
6. Taher AT, Musallam KM, Nasreddine W, et al. Asymptomatic brain magnetic resonance imaging abnormalities in splenectomized adults with thalassemia intermedia. J Thromb Haemost. 2010;8:54-9.
7. Vasilopoulou M, Stafylidis C, Politou M. The thrombotic spectrum of Β-thalassemia: Thrombosis Update. 2022;7:100102.
8. Taher AT, Otrock ZK, Uthman I, et al. Thalassemia and hypercoagulability; Blood Rev. 2008;22(5):283-92.
9. Hashemieh M. Thromboembolic events in severe thalassemia syndromes. IJBC. 2020;12(2):41-6.
10. Bahrani S, Teimouri-jervekani Z, Sadeghi M. Thrombotic events and anticoagulants in beta-thalassemia patients with focus on anticoagulants for atrial fibrillation: a brief review. Curr Probl Cardiol. 2021;47(9):100912.
11. Taher AT, Cappellini MD, Musallam KM. Development of a thalassemia-related thrombosis risk scoring system. Am J Hematol. 2019;94(8):E207-9.
12. Taher A, Isma'eel H, Cappellini MD. Thalassemia intermedia: revisited. Blood Cells Mol Dis. 2006;37(1):12-20.
13. Musallam KM, Rivella S, Vichinsky E, et al. Non-transfusion-dependent thalassemias. Haematologica. 2013;98(6):833-44.
14. Olivieri NF, Muraca GM, O'Donnell A, et al. Studies in haemoglobin E beta-thalassaemia. Br J Haematol. 2008;141(3):388-97.
15. Mehta V, Kirubarajan A, Sabouhanian A, et al. Leg Ulcers: A Report in Patients with Hemoglobin E Beta Thalassemia and Review of the Literature in Severe Beta Thalassemia. Acta Haematol. 2022;145(3):334-43.
16. Musallam KM, Taher AT, Duca L, et al. Levels of growth differentiation factor-15 are high and correlate with clinical severity in transfusion-independent patients with beta thalassemia intermedia. Blood Cells Mol Dis. 2011;47(4):232-4.
17. Musallam KM, Taher AT, Rachmilewitz EA. beta-thalassemia intermedia: a clinical perspective. Cold Spring Harb Perspect Med. 2012;2(7):a013482.
18. Matta BN, Abbas O, Maakaron JE, et al. Leg ulcers in patients with beta-thalassaemia intermedia: a single centre's experience. J Eur Acad Dermatol Venereol. 2014;28(9):1245-50.
19. Musallam KM, Cappellini MD, Daar S, et al. Morbidity-free survival and hemoglobin level in non-transfusion-dependent beta-thalassemia: a 10-year cohort study. Ann Hematol. 2022; 101(1):203-4.
20. Taher AT, Musallam KM, Saliba AN, et al. Hemoglobin level and morbidity in non-transfusion-dependent thalassemia. Blood Cells Mol Dis. 2015;55(2):108-9.
21. Opartkiattikul N, Sukpanichnant S, Wanachiwanawin W, et al. A double-blind placebo control trial of dilazep in beta-thalassemia/hemoglobin E patients. Southeast Asian J Trop Med Public Health. 1997;28 Suppl 3:167-71.
22. Minniti CP, Gorbach AM, Xu D, et al. Topical sodium nitrite for chronic leg ulcers in patients with sickle cell anaemia: a phase 1 dose-finding safety and tolerability trial. Lancet Haematol. 2014;1(3):e95-e103.
23. Piga A, Perrotta S, Gamberini MR, et al. Luspatercept improves hemoglobin levels and blood transfusion requirements in a study of patients with beta-thalassemia. Blood. 2019;133(12):1279-89.
24. Winichakoon P, Tantiworawit A, Rattanathammethee T, et al. Prevalence and Risk Factors for Complications in Patients with Nontransfusion Dependent Alpha- and Beta-Thalassemia. Anemia. 2015;2015:793025
25. Lotfi M, Keramati P, Assdsangabi R, et al. Ultrasonographic assessment of the prevalence of cholelithiasis and biliary sludge in beta-thalassemia patients in Iran. Med Sci Monit. 2009;15(8):CR398-402.
26. Galanello R, Piras S, Barella S, et al. Cholelithiasis and Gilbert's syndrome in homozygous β-thalassaemia. Br J Haematol. 2001;115(4):926-8.
27. Sherlock S, Dooley J. Diseases of the liver and biliary system. Gut. 2003;52(4):615.
28. Mishra AK, Tiwari A. Iron overload in beta thalassaemia major and intermedia patients. Maedica (Buchar). 2013;8(4):328-32.

29. Khavari M, Hamidi A, Haghpanah S, et al. Frequency of Cholelithiasis in Patients with Beta-Thalassemia Intermedia with and without Hydroxyurea. Iran Red Crescent Med J. 2014;16(7):e18712.
30. Portincasa P, Moschetta A, Berardino M, et al. Impaired gallbladder motility and delayed orocecal transit contribute to pigment gallstone and biliary sludge formation in beta-thalassemia major adults. World J Gastroenterol. 2004;10(16):2383-90.
31. Shahramian I, Behzadmehr R, Afshari M, et al. Cholelithiasis in Thalassemia Major Patients: A Report from the South-East of Iran. Int J Hematol Oncol Stem Cell Res. 2018;12(2):117-22.

13 CHAPTER

Evaluation of Cardiac Status in Thalassemia

Sudha Sethy, Amiya Ranjan Nayak

INTRODUCTION

Cardiovascular complications remain a major cause of morbidity and mortality in β-thalassemia despite advances in management. Limited access to optimal therapies, poor compliance, and age-related issues contribute to this burden. MRI-guided chelation has improved survival, but access disparities persist, especially in low- and middle-income countries (LMICs). Cardiac complications are observed in 42% and contribute to 71% of all deaths in transfusion-dependent thalassemia (TDT) patients.[1]

PATHOPHYSIOLOGY (SUMMARIZED IN FLOWCHART 1)

In β-thalassemia, persistent hemolysis and ineffective erythropoiesis result in chronic anemia, prompting compensatory bone marrow expansion and elevated fetal hemoglobin (HbF) production. Despite these adaptations, oxygen delivery remains inadequate, leading to high-output heart failure as the heart works harder to meet metabolic demands.[2] Patients require frequent blood transfusions, which, along with increased gastrointestinal iron

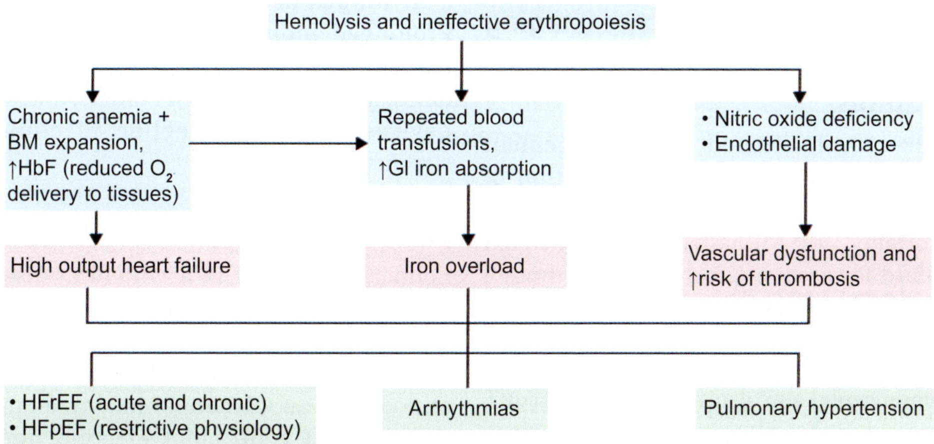

FLOWCHART 1: Pathophysiology of major cardiovascular complications in thalassemia.
(BM: bone marrow; HbF: hemoglobin F; O_2: oxygen; GI: gastrointestinal; HFrEF: heart failure with reduced ejection fraction; HFpEF: heart failure with preserved ejection fraction)

absorption, contribute to systemic iron overload.

Within cardiomyocytes, iron is initially stored in ferritin. However, when storage capacity is exceeded, excess free iron accumulates, generating oxidative stress and causing cellular toxicity, ultimately impairing myocardial function. Importantly, cardiac iron overload may remain clinically silent for years before manifesting as acute cardiac decompensation, often triggered by infections or metabolic stressors.[3] Additionally, chronic hemolysis leads to nitric oxide depletion, contributing to endothelial dysfunction, vascular injury, and an elevated risk of thrombosis.[4]

All these events increase the risk of heart failure with reduced ejection fraction (HFrEF) due to direct myocardial injury and heart failure with preserved ejection fraction (HFpEF) resulting from restrictive physiology and diastolic dysfunction. Additionally, risk of pulmonary hypertension also increases substantially. Splenectomy further exacerbates risk of thrombosis and pulmonary hypertension.[5]

DIAGNOSTIC CARDIAC EVALUATION

Cardiac Magnetic Resonance Imaging (Gold Standard for Assessing Cardiac Iron Status)

MRI has revolutionized TDT management by enabling noninvasive quantification of tissue iron, contributing to a 70% reduction in mortality.[6] T2* MRI at 1.5 Tesla is the gold standard for assessing cardiac iron, though accuracy depends on strict adherence to scanning protocols. Iron content is quantified using relaxation parameters, primarily R2* and T2*. T2* is the reciprocal of R2* (T2* = 1/R2*), meaning that as iron concentration increases, R2* rises while T2* declines. A falling T2* indicates rising cardiac iron and increased heart failure risk. Studies using cardiovascular magnetic resonance (CMR) imaging have demonstrated a strong, graded relationship between myocardial iron load (T2* <20 ms) and left ventricular ejection fraction (LVEF) decline, highlighting its prognostic value.[7]

Cardiac MRI T2* assessment should be conducted alongside hepatic MRI T2* at intervals based on the patient's iron burden and local guidelines. Generally, the first MRI T2* scan is recommended 8 years after starting blood transfusions and is subsequently repeated every 2 years.[8] Annual monitoring is required in patients with established cardiac dysfunction (T2* <20 ms or heart disease). For T2* <10 ms, 6 monthly monitoring is advised.[9]

Despite its critical role, MRI accessibility in many parts of India remains limited due to cost and complexity. Where MRI availability is limited, prioritize scans for patients aged 10–18 years with SF > 2,500 ng/mL, followed by any patient with SF > 2,500 ng/mL, to optimize chelation and prevent complications.[9]

Electrocardiogram

The ECG is essential in cardiovascular assessment but may miss intermittent arrhythmias or myocardial iron overload. Prolonged monitoring options, including Holter monitors, wearable patches (7–14 days), implantable loop recorders, and smart devices, improve detection of clinically significant events.[10]

Echocardiography

Echocardiography is a widely accessible, safe, and non-invasive tool that enables real-time bedside cardiovascular assessment. Assessment includes chamber size evaluation and detection of congenital or acquired defects. Left ventricular ejection fraction (LVEF) is the most commonly used measure of systolic function, but its reliability improves with advanced techniques like 3D/4D volumetric analysis. Since LVEF declines late in iron overload, early myocardial dysfunction is better detected using tissue Doppler imaging (TDI) and global longitudinal strain (GLS).[11] Echocardiography is also essential for pulmonary hypertension screening, with a tricuspid valve regurgitant jet velocity (TRVmax) >3.2 m/s indicating high risk. Early referral is crucial to prevent irreversible vascular changes.[12]

When MRI is unavailable, ECG, echocardiography, and clinical examination become crucial for assessing cardiac status. These assessments should be conducted annually, with the frequency increased to every 3–6 months if cardiac disease is detected.[5]

Blood Biomarkers

Cardiac biomarkers like NT-proBNP and troponin have a limited role in routine iron overload management but are valuable for assessing acute decompensation and monitoring heart failure.[13] NT-proBNP can also enhance pulmonary hypertension screening accuracy.

Cardiac Catheterization

When echocardiographic findings are inconclusive, invasive right heart catheterization is necessary for definitive pulmonary hypertension diagnosis. A mean pulmonary arterial pressure >25 mm Hg at rest confirms the condition. Catheterization is typically reserved for suspected pre-capillary pulmonary hypertension when considering targeted pulmonary arterial hypertension therapies.[14]

MANAGEMENT OF SPECIFIC ISSUES

Acute Decompensated Heart Failure

The primary goal in managing acute heart failure due to iron overload is stabilization and initiation of continuous iron chelation therapy. Immediate treatment includes IV deferoxamine (50 mg/kg/day) and early introduction of deferiprone (75 mg/kg/day in divided doses). Continuous ECG and hemodynamic monitoring, along with bedside echocardiography, are essential to confirm heart failure and rule out other conditions. Hemodynamic support should maintain cerebral and renal perfusion while avoiding aggressive inotropic therapy. Minimal diuretics are recommended to preserve preload, with venous ultrafiltration as an alternative. Arrhythmia management involves correcting electrolytes, using magnesium infusion for ventricular arrhythmias, and amiodarone for hemodynamically significant cases. β-blockers may be introduced if stable. Additional measures include glucose control, hydrocortisone for adrenal insufficiency, and correction of metabolic imbalances. Hemoglobin should be maintained at 10–12 g/dL with small transfusions(5–10 mL/kg), and infections or other triggers should be promptly addressed.

Cardiac MRI T2* should be performed as soon as possible to assess myocardial iron content. If T2* is >20 ms, myocarditis should be considered and evaluated using an MRI protocol. While stabilization may take weeks to months, early dialysis may be needed for patients with renal failure to remove the iron-chelator complex. Deferasirox is generally avoided due to concerns over renal perfusion. Mechanical support devices for ventricular support may be considered, though evidence is limited. If the initial treatment response is inadequate, early consultation with a transplant center is recommended.[13]

Chronic HFrEF

Patients with myocardial iron overload and a declining or abnormal LVEF, even if asymptomatic, are at risk of early heart failure. Consistent monitoring using imaging techniques like CMR or echocardiography is crucial. Tracking LVEF and cardiac dimensions helps assess treatment response, with worsening function signaling the need for more aggressive therapy. Randomized trials indicate that deferoxamine alone does not significantly enhance LVEF in mild to moderate cardiac iron overload, whereas addition of deferiprone has shown notable benefits.[15,16] Origa et al. observed a significant improvement in LVEF, rising from 49 ± 9% to 57 ± 1% ($p = 0.001$), in a cohort of 20 patients receiving combination therapy.[17] An increase in LVEF suggests relief from subclinical cardiotoxicity and a reduced risk of heart failure. If cardiac function fails to improve, other potential contributors, such as cardiomyopathy, should be considered. While cardiac T2* trends may provide prognostic insight, in settings where CMR is unavailable, serial cardiac function assessments remain vital for detecting heart failure risk.

HFpEF

Cardiac restriction in β-thalassemia is characterized by reduced ventricular compliance, leading to increased diastolic filling pressures and atrial enlargement. While systolic function is often preserved initially, abnormalities in longitudinal function and progressive diastolic dysfunction can eventually lead to systolic impairment.[18] Chronic iron overload, anemia-induced high-output states, vascular dysfunction, and diabetes contribute to this pathology, increasing the risk of HFpEF and right-sided heart failure due to pulmonary hypertension.

Patients experience fluid congestion, edema, hepatic congestion, exercise intolerance, and a high risk of atrial fibrillation. Historically, treatment focused on symptom management with diuretics, but SGLT2 inhibitors have now shown mortality benefits across all heart failure types, including HFpEF. Though specific data in β-thalassemia is lacking, early introduction of SGLT2i may be beneficial. Prevention remains key, emphasizing optimal hemoglobin levels, intensive iron chelation, and early SGLT2i use in patients with diabetes or CKD to reduce heart failure risk.[19]

Arrhythmias

Arrhythmias are common in iron-loaded patients, with atrial fibrillation (AF) being the most frequent.[20] The risk increases with age and depends on cardiac iron load and ventricular function. Severe iron overload can cause life-threatening arrhythmias, including complete heart block (CHB) and ventricular tachycardia, necessitating urgent intervention. While CHB may reverse with intensive deferoxamine chelation, pacemaker implantation is often required. Ventricular tachycardia, linked to severe iron overload, carries a high risk of sudden death and may require hospitalization and an implantable cardioverter-defibrillator (ICD), along with aggressive iron chelation.

In younger β-thalassemia patients, AF is usually linked to iron overload and can trigger acute decompensation, requiring urgent cardioversion and chelation. In older patients (>40 years), AF is often unrelated to iron levels and associated with diabetes, prior iron overload, and ECG abnormalities like right bundle branch block. Up to 40% of β-thalassemia patients over 40 develop AF, increasing embolism risk, especially post-splenectomy.[21] Standard stroke risk calculators are unreliable in these patients, so anticoagulation decisions should be individualized. Management includes optimizing iron levels, cardiac function, and comorbidities, with advanced interventions like ablation or pacemaker therapy for refractory cases.

Pulmonary Hypertension

Pulmonary hypertension (PH) is uncommon in TDT (~0.8% in Europe) but more prevalent in NTDT, particularly among splenectomized adults and in low- and middle-income countries (LMICs).[22] A study from a tertiary care hospital in India reported PAH in 31.6% of TDT patients, highlighting the higher prevalence in LMICs.[23] PH due to left ventricular dysfunction (HFpEF/HFrEF) requires early intervention with iron chelation, optimal hemoglobin maintenance, standard heart failure therapy, and possibly SGLT2 inhibitors. Pulmonary arterial hypertension (PAH), more commonly seen in under-transfused patients, is associated with chronic hemolysis and has a poor prognosis, with a 5-year survival rate of approximately 60%.[14]

PH in β-thalassemia is linked to factors such as NTDT, suboptimal transfusion in TDT, splenectomy, thrombocytosis (≥500 × 10^9/L), elevated nRBC count (≥300 × 10^6/L), hemoglobin < 9 g/dL, significant iron overload, and a history of thrombosis. Annual echocardiographic assessment of tricuspid regurgitation velocity (TRV) is recommended, with close monitoring for asymptomatic cases (TRV 2.5–3.2 m/s) and right heart catheterization for symptomatic or high TRV cases (>3.2 m/s). Management includes regular transfusions, hydroxycarbamide, iron chelation, anticoagulation in select cases, and cardiology-guided treatment per PHT guidelines.[20]

Other Forms of Cardiovascular Disease

Thromboembolism

The hypercoagulable state in β-thalassemia increases the risk of arterial and venous thrombosis, with NTDT patients facing a fourfold higher risk than those with TDT.[24] This heightened risk is driven by factors such as hemolyzed red cell-induced thrombogenicity, platelet activation, thrombocytosis, iron-related endothelial damage, and coagulopathy, particularly in splenectomized adults.[25] Strokes, even in younger patients, are increasingly recognized, with atrial fibrillation playing a major role.

Thrombotic disease in β-thalassemia is managed per standard guidelines, with additional thrombophilia screening for unprovoked or unusual-site thrombosis. Risk stratification and prophylaxis are individualized due to the lack of specific data, with high-risk patients—including NTDT, splenectomized individuals, and those with low hemoglobin or high platelet counts—often receiving enoxaparin or newer oral anticoagulants. Blood transfusions help reduce thrombotic risk in NTDT by improving erythropoiesis and lowering thrombogenic cells, though no standardized transfusion protocol exists. Aspirin is routinely given to splenectomized patients, as studies suggest it may reduce thrombotic recurrence.[26]

Pericarditis and Myocarditis

Acute pericarditis was once common in poorly managed thalassemia major (TM), affecting nearly half of patients before the advent of regular therapy in the 1960s. Improved management of anemia, iron overload, and transfusion quality has significantly reduced its occurrence, with a reported prevalence of 5% in well-treated TM patients and 8% in nontransfused thalassemia intermedia (TI) patients.[27] Similarly, acute myocarditis was observed in 4% of TM patients over a decade, with histopathological confirmation in half of the cases. It led to left ventricular dysfunction in 23%, chronic heart failure in 28%, and ventricular tachycardia in 9%. However, advancements in anemia and iron overload management have significantly lowered its incidence.[28]

Valvular Disease

Valvular abnormalities, including calcification, mild to moderate mitral and tricuspid regurgitation, and mitral valve prolapse, are relatively common in patients with haemoglobinopathies, especially those with untreated or poorly managed NTDT cases.[28]

CONCLUSION

Cardiovascular (CV) disease has been the leading cause of mortality in thalassemia but has significantly declined with modern multidisciplinary care. Its pathophysiology and presentation vary based on disease interactions and treatment approaches. Iron overload cardiomyopathy, once the primary cardiac complication in transfusion-treated patients, is now effectively prevented with MRI-guided chelation therapy. Regular CV assessment should be integrated into multidisciplinary monitoring, ideally involving specialists in hemoglobinopathy-related heart disease. Prevention and treatment rely not only on cardioactive therapies but also on optimizing disease-specific management and addressing comorbidities. A heart-healthy lifestyle is essential, and early intervention can potentially reverse cardiac dysfunction and heart failure.

SUMMARY AND RECOMMENDATIONS

1. Use Cardiac MRI T2* as the gold standard for assessing myocardial iron. Begin screening 8 years after transfusions start and repeat every 2 years; increase to annually or 6-monthly if T2* <20 ms or cardiac dysfunction is present respectively.
2. Prioritize MRI in settings with limited access for:
   - Patients aged 10–18 years with SF > 2,500 ng/mL
   - Any patient with SF > 2,500 ng/mL
   - Patients with rising SF despite chelation
3. Conduct annual ECG and echocardiography for cardiac monitoring, with increased frequency (every 3–6 months) in those with known cardiac disease or when MRI is unavailable.
4. Use advanced echocardiographic techniques (TDI, GLS, 3D echo) to detect early myocardial dysfunction, as LVEF may remain preserved in early stages of cardiac iron overload.
5. Employ cardiac biomarkers (NT-proBNP, troponin) for acute heart failure assessment and pulmonary hypertension risk stratification—not for routine monitoring.
6. Confirm pulmonary hypertension with right heart catheterization if echocardiographic findings are inconclusive or if TRVmax > 3.2 m/s.
7. Manage acute decompensated heart failure with:
   - IV deferoxamine + deferiprone
   - Gentle hemodynamic support and minimal diuretics
   - ECG, echocardiography, and cardiac MRI
   - Early referral if poor response to chelation
8. Initiate combination chelation therapy (e.g., deferiprone + deferoxamine) in chronic HFrEF with cardiac iron overload; monitor LVEF to guide therapy escalation.
9. Treat HFpEF with optimal chelation, anemia control, and early use of SGLT2 inhibitors, especially in patients with diabetes or CKD.
10. Screen and manage arrhythmias and thromboembolic risk proactively:
    - Monitor for AF, CHB, and VT in iron-overloaded patients
    - Use individualized anticoagulation, especially postsplenectomy or in patients with high TRV or AF
    - Address reversible causes, and consider pacemakers or ICDs for high-risk arrhythmias

REFERENCES

1. Koohi F, Kazemi T, Miri-Moghaddam E. Cardiac complications and iron overload in beta thalassemia major patients-a systematic review and meta-analysis. Ann Hematol. 2019;98(6):1323-31.
2. Aessopos A, Farmakis D, Deftereos S, et al. Thalassemia heart disease: a comparative evaluation of thalassemia major and thalassemia intermedia. Chest. 2005;127:1523-30.
3. Kremastinos DT, Farmakis D. Iron overload cardiomyopathy in clinical practice. Circulation. 2011;124:2253-63.
4. Cheung YF, Chan GC, Ha SY. Arterial stiffness and endothelial function in patients with beta-thalassemia major. Circulation. 2002;106:2561-6
5. Farmakis D, Triposkiadis F, Lekakis J, et al. Heart failure in haemoglobinopathies: pathophysiology, clinical phenotypes, and management. Eur J Heart Fail. 2017;19(4):479-89.
6. Modell B, Khan M, Darlison M, et al. Improved survival of thalassaemia major in the UK and relation to T2* cardiovascular magnetic resonance. J Cardiovasc Magn Reson. 2008;10(1):42.
7. Alam MH, Auger D, McGill LA, et al. Comparison of 3 T and 1.5 T for T2* magnetic resonance of tissue iron. J Cardiovasc Magn Reson. 2016;18(1):40.
8. Abdel-Gadir A, Vorasettakarnkij Y, Ngamkasem H, et al. Ultrafast Magnetic Resonance Imaging for Iron Quantification in Thalassemia Participants in the Developing World: The TIC-TOC Study (Thailand and UK International Collaboration in Thalassaemia Optimising Ultrafast CMR). Circulation. 2016;134(5):432-4.
9. Viprakasit V, Ajlan A, Aydinok Y, et al. MRI for the diagnosis of cardiac and liver iron overload in patients with transfusion-dependent thalassemia: An algorithm to guide clinical use when availability is limited. Am J Hematol. 2018;93(6):E135-7.
10. Steinberg JS, Varma N, Cygankiewicz I, et al. 2017 ISHNE-HRS expert consensus statement on ambulatory ECG and external cardiac monitoring/telemetry. Heart Rhythm. 2018;15(5):789.
11. Fianza PI, Pramono AA, Ghozali M, et al. Diagnostic Modalities in Detecting Cardiovascular Complications of Thalassemia. Rev Cardiovasc Med. 2022;23(8):267.
12. Derchi G, Musallam KM, Pinto VM, et al. Tricuspid-valve regurgitant jet velocity as a risk factor for death in β-thalassemia. Haematologica. 2022;107(7):1714-8.
13. Pennell DJ, Udelson JE, Arai AE, et al. Cardiovascular function and treatment in β-thalassemia major: a consensus statement from the American Heart Association. Circulation. 2013;128(3):281-308.
14. Pinto VM, Musallam KM, Derchi G, et al. Mortality in β-thalassemia patients with confirmed pulmonary arterial hypertension on right heart catheterization. Blood. 2022;139(13):2080-3.
15. Galanello R, Agus A, Campus S, et al. Combined iron chelation therapy. Ann Ny Acad Sci. 2010;1202(1):79-86.
16. Tanner MA, Galanello R, Dessi C, et al. Combined chelation therapy in thalassemia major for the treatment of severe myocardial siderosis with left ventricular dysfunction. J Cardiovasc Magn Reson. 2008;10(1):12.
17. Origa R, Bina P, Agus A, et al. Combined therapy with deferiprone and desferrioxamine in thalassemia major. Haematologica. 2005;90:1309-14.
18. Vogel M, Anderson LJ, Holden S, et al. Tissue Doppler echocardiography in patients with thalassaemia detects early myocardial dysfunction related to myocardial iron overload. Eur Heart J. 2003;24(1):113-9.
19. McDonagh TA, Metra M, Adamo M, et al. 2021 ESC Guidelines for the diagnosis and treatment of acute and chronic heart failure [published correction appears in Eur Heart J. 2021;42(48):4901.
20. Taher AT, Cappellini MD. How I manage medical complications of beta-thalassemia in adults. Blood. 2018;132(17):1781-91.
21. Bell RM, Mohamed S, Ako EA, et al. The prevalence and risk factors for atrial fibrillation in beta-thalassemia major: a cross-sectional study in a UK specialist cardio-haematology clinic. Eur Heart J. 2015;36(12):916.
22. Derchi G, Galanello R, Bina P, et al. Prevalence and risk factors for pulmonary arterial hypertension in a large group of β-thalassemia patients using right heart catheterization: a Webthal study. Circulation. 2014;129(3):338-45.
23. Gupta V, Vijayakumar V, Aggarwal P, et al. Pulmonary Artery Hypertension in Transfusion-Dependent Thalassemia. Indian Pediatr. 2024;61(1):49-52.
24. Taher A, Isma'eel H, Mehio G, et al. Prevalence of thromboembolic events among 8,860 patients with thalassaemia major and intermedia in the

Mediterranean area and Iran. Thromb Haemost. 2006;96(4):488-91.
25. Eldor A, Rachmilewitz EA. The hypercoagulable state in thalassemia. Blood. 2002;99(1):36-43.
26. Taher AT, Cappellini MD, Musallam KM. Development of a thalassemia-related thrombosis risk scoring system. Am J Hematol. 2019;4(8):E207-9.
27. Aessopos A, Farmakis D, Karagiorga M, et al. Cardiac involvement in thalassemia intermedia: a multicenter study. Blood. 2001;97(11):3411-6.
28. Kremastinos DT, Tiniakos G, Theodorakis GN, et al. Myocarditis in β-thalassemia major: a cause of heart failure. Circulation. 1995;91:66-71.

14

CHAPTER

Endocrine Evaluation in Thalassemia

Sujoy Ghosh

INTRODUCTION

Endocrine dysfunctions are among the most frequent and significant complications observed in patients with transfusion-dependent thalassemia. Chronic anemia, hypoxia, and iron overload—particularly in the pituitary, thyroid, adrenal, and gonadal tissues—contribute to the development of multiple endocrine abnormalities. Early identification and systematic evaluation of growth failure, hypogonadism, hypothyroidism, adrenal insufficiency, hypoparathyroidism, diabetes, and bone disease are crucial for improving long-term outcomes and quality of life. This chapter outlines a stepwise approach to endocrine assessment in thalassemia using flowcharts, highlighting clinical, biochemical, and imaging criteria for diagnosis and management.

GROWTH FAILURE[1-4]

Growth should be evaluated using the combined WHO-IAP growth charts to ensure accurate assessment based on age and gender. Short stature is defined as height below the third centile for age and gender or a height velocity below 1 SD for age and gender over 1 year. Immediate evaluation for growth failure is indicated if height is more than 3 SD below the mean for chronological age, more than 1.5 SD below the mid-parental height, or more than 2 SD below the mean with a height velocity over 1 SD below the mean for 1 year. Additionally, height velocity more than 2 SD below the mean over 1 year or sustained more than 1.5 SD below the mean over 2 years also warrants investigation. The mid-parental height should be calculated as (father's height + mother's height)/2 + 6.5 cm for boys and (father's height + mother's height)/2–6.5 cm for girls. Bone age estimation by X-ray of the left hand including the wrist joint is advised if auxologic parameters indicate short stature. If a child meets the criteria for short stature, serum IGF-1 should be measured. A low IGF-1 for chronological age necessitates referral to an endocrinologist for confirmation of growth hormone (GH) deficiency using GH stimulation tests. The insulin tolerance test is considered the gold standard, while the glucagon stimulation test is preferred for its safety; the clonidine test is another alternative. A peak GH level < 7 μg/L with glucagon stimulation confirms GH deficiency. MRI of the hypothalamo-pituitary region is not routinely required in thalassemia patients unless GH deficiency is proven. Management includes optimizing blood transfusion, nutrition, and iron chelation. In confirmed GH deficiency, recombinant human growth hormone (rhGH) may be used off-label under specialist care, at a dose between 0.17 and 0.33 mg/kg/week, most commonly 0.2 mg/kg/week. Serum IGF-1 should be monitored at least annually during rhGH therapy. The stepwise approach for growth assessment is shown in **Flowchart 1**.

HYPOGONADISM[5-10]

Absence of secondary sexual characteristics, menstrual irregularities such as amenorrhea or oligomenorrhea, erectile dysfunction, gynecomastia, and infertility are clinical indicators of hypogonadism. The earliest sign of puberty in males is testicular enlargement to ≥4 mL, assessed using a Prader orchidometer, while in females, the first sign is growth spurt and breast bud development. A profile showing low gonadal hormones with low or inappropriately normal LH and FSH levels indicates hypogonadotropic hypogonadism, whereas low testosterone or estradiol with elevated LH and FSH levels suggests primary (gonadal) hypogonadism. In uncertain cases, an endocrinologist should be consulted for a GnRH stimulation test, where a post-GnRH agonist stimulated LH <5 mIU/mL after 3 hours confirms hypogonadism. MRI of the hypothalamo-pituitary (HP) region is recommended when hormonal evaluation suggests hypogonadotropic hypogonadism, with pituitary height <4.4 mm serving as a predictor. MRI surveillance is especially critical between 10–20 years of age, when pituitary iron accumulation is most rapid. In females, pelvic ultrasonography should be performed to assess ovarian volume, uterine length, and endometrial thickness. In boys with confirmed hypogonadism, testosterone enanthate or cypionate should be initiated at 50 mg intramuscularly once a month from 14 years of age under specialist supervision, with gradual escalation to an adult dose of 250 mg every 3–4 weeks over 3–4 years. For girls, low-dose 17-beta estradiol (0.25 mg orally) should begin at 13 years of age, with the dose gradually increased to 2 mg daily over 24 months. Cyclical progestin therapy should be added after 2 years of estradiol therapy or once breakthrough bleeding occurs. Pubertal induction using combination therapy with hCG and recombinant FSH may also be considered based on patient preference and clinical guidance. The stepwise assessment is detailed in **Flowchart 2**.

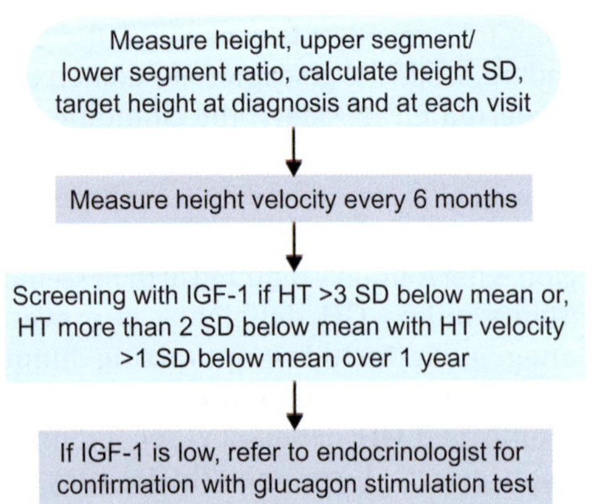

FLOWCHART 1: Stepwise approach to growth failure in patients with thalassemia.

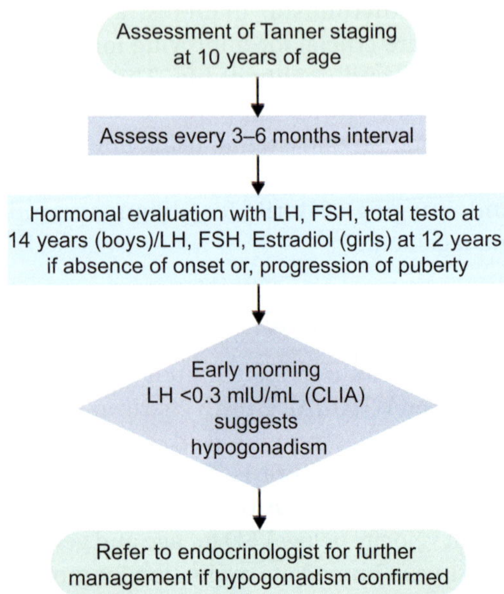

FLOWCHART 2: Stepwise approach for assessment of hypogonadism.

ADRENAL DYSFUNCTION[11-14]

The stepwise approach for assessing adrenal insufficiency is detailed in **Flowchart 3**. Primary adrenal insufficiency is diagnosed when serum cortisol is less than 5 µg/dL along with adrenocorticotropic hormone (ACTH) levels more than twice the upper normal limit. Since ACTH is a heat-labile peptide, it must be collected in a prechilled EDTA vial and delivered to the laboratory within 5–10 minutes of collection to ensure accuracy. This condition is typically associated with low aldosterone levels, elevated plasma renin activity (PRA) or direct renin concentration (DRC), hyponatremia, and hyperkalemia. In contrast, secondary adrenal insufficiency is characterized by low cortisol with low or inappropriately normal ACTH levels and is usually associated with normal aldosterone, PRA/DRC, and electrolyte levels. The ACTH stimulation test is employed to confirm adrenal insufficiency in patients with borderline cortisol levels (5–10 µg/dL). In this test, 250 µg of cosyntropin is administered intravenously, and cortisol levels are measured at 30 and 60 minutes. A peak cortisol response below 18.1 µg/dL confirms the diagnosis of adrenal insufficiency.

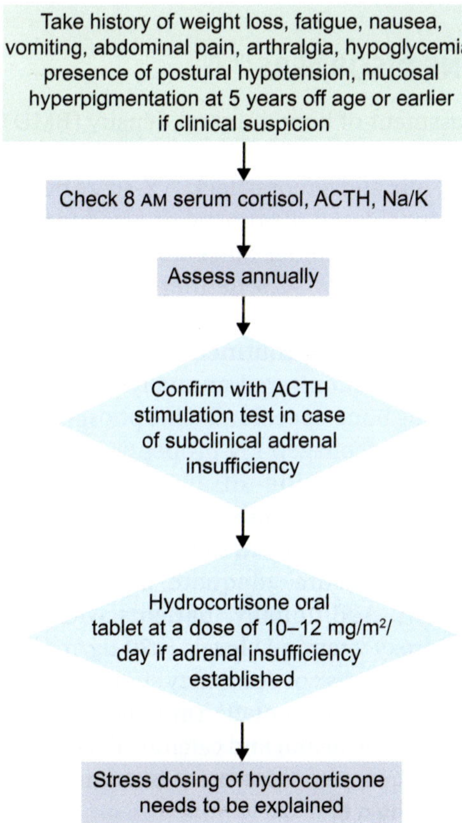

FLOWCHART 3: Stepwise approach for assessing adrenal dysfunction.

HYPOTHYROIDISM[15,16]

Assessment for hypothyroidism is detailed in **Flowchart 4**. The dose of levothyroxine varies according to age: 4 µg/kg/day for children aged 6–12 years, 3 µg/kg/day for those older than 12 years, and 1.6–1.8 µg/kg/day for postpubertal individuals. Before initiating levothyroxine therapy, it is essential to rule

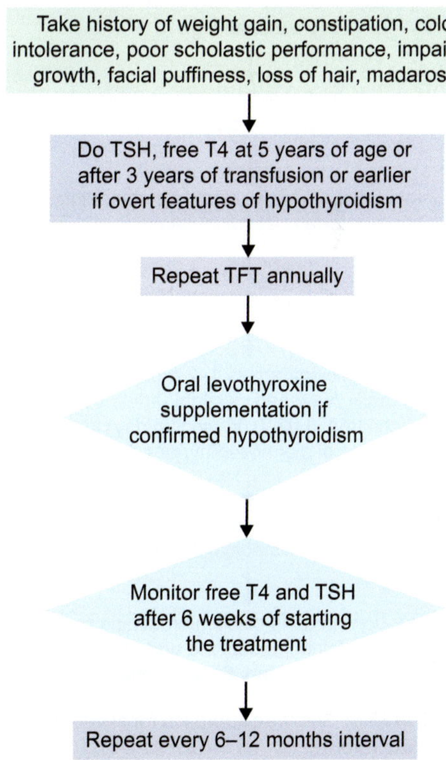

FLOWCHART 4: Stepwise approach for assessment of thyroid function.

out underlying cortisol deficiency to prevent adrenal crisis. An elevated TSH with decreased T4 indicates primary hypothyroidism, whereas low or inappropriately normal TSH with decreased T4 suggests secondary hypothyroidism. During treatment, TSH should be maintained within the mid-normal reference range in primary hypothyroidism, while in secondary hypothyroidism, free T4 (FT4) should be kept in the upper half of the normal reference range to ensure adequate hormone replacement.

HYPOPARATHYROIDISM[17,18]

Clinical and lab assessment for hypoparathyroidism is detailed in **Flowchart 5**.

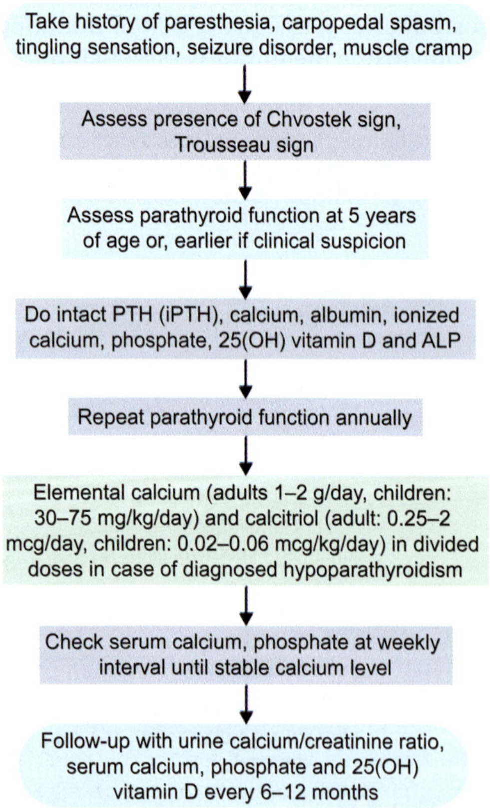

FLOWCHART 5: Stepwise approach for assessment of hypoparathyroidism.

Hypoparathyroidism may often be asymptomatic, though in some cases, a prolonged QT interval on ECG can serve as an indicator of underlying hypocalcemia. It is characterized by low serum calcium levels accompanied by low or inappropriately normal serum intact parathyroid hormone (PTH) concentrations. Most patients with hypoparathyroidism also exhibit elevated serum phosphorus levels due to impaired PTH-mediated phosphate excretion. For management, various calcium preparations such as calcium citrate, calcium carbonate, and calcium gluconate are available and can be used depending on clinical context and patient tolerance. The goal of therapy is to maintain serum calcium between 8 and 8.5 mg/dL to achieve symptom control while preventing hypercalciuria and its renal complications.

BONE DISORDERS[19,20]

Assessment of bone mineral density (BMD) should include measurement at the lumbar spine, hip, and femoral neck. A Z-score below –2 is considered diagnostic of osteoporosis in individuals under 50 years of age, while a T-score below –2.5 defines osteoporosis in those above 50 years. Bone turnover markers are not routinely recommended but may be monitored annually if feasible, including bone-specific alkaline phosphatase (bALP), Procollagen I N-propeptide (PINP), and C-telopeptide of type I collagen (CTX). Calcium supplementation of up to 1,300 mg/day is advised starting from 9 years of age to ensure adequate bone mineralization. Additionally, patients with low 25-hydroxy vitamin D levels (<30 ng/mL) or those at high risk of deficiency should receive vitamin D supplementation at 1,000 IU/day to support bone health and calcium absorption. The frequency of assessment is summarized in **Flowchart 6**.

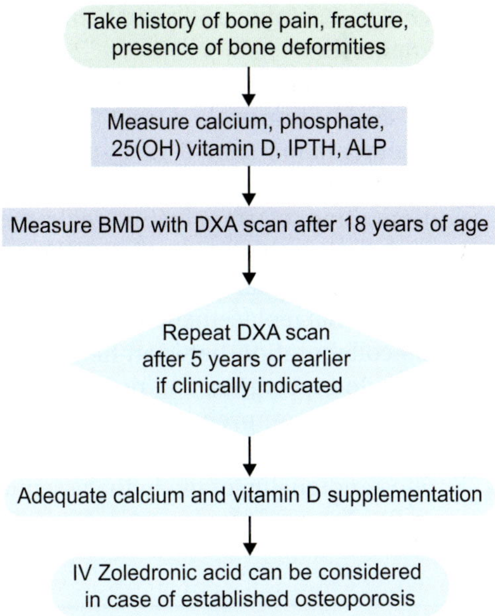

FLOWCHART 6: Stepwise approach for assessing bone status.

DIABETES[21,22]

The assessment for diabetes mellitus is detailed in **Flowchart 7**. The diagnosis and management are the same as in patients with diabetes mellitus without thalassemia. HbA1c cannot be used in diagnosis as well as in follow-up in thalassemia, as it is falsely low in most of the situations due to shortened RBC life span and elevated fetal Hb.

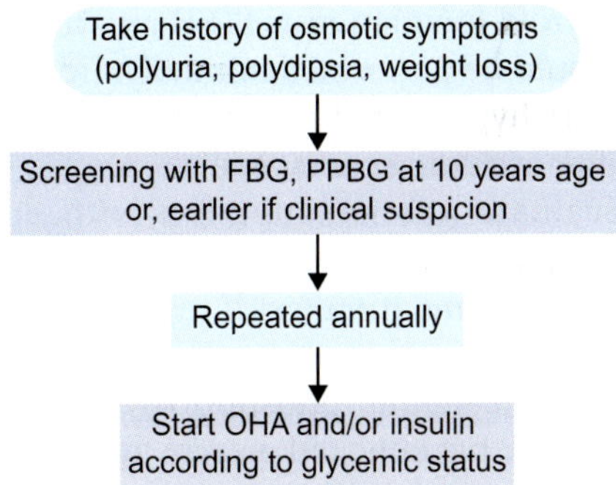

FLOWCHART 7: Stepwise approach for assessment of diabetes.

CONCLUSION

Comprehensive endocrine evaluation is an essential component of long-term care in patients with thalassemia. Regular, structured screening helps in timely detection and treatment of hormonal deficiencies, thereby preventing irreversible complications. Optimization of transfusion, iron chelation, and nutritional support forms the foundation of endocrine health in thalassemia. Collaboration between hematologists and endocrinologists is key to ensuring individualized, evidence-based management and improving overall survival and quality of life.

SUMMARY OF RECOMMENDATIONS

- Endocrine dysfunction is a common long-term complication in transfusion-dependent thalassemia, primarily due to chronic iron overload and pituitary iron deposition.
- Annual screening for growth, pubertal status, thyroid, adrenal, calcium, and bone health should begin from early childhood in all thalassemia patients.
- Growth should be monitored using WHO-IAP combined growth charts, and bone age assessment performed if short stature or poor height velocity is noted.
- Serum IGF-1 measurement is the first step in evaluating growth failure; if low, refer to an endocrinologist for GH stimulation testing to confirm growth hormone deficiency.
- Pubertal assessment is critical—absence or delay in secondary sexual characteristics warrants evaluation for hypogonadotropic or primary hypogonadism with LH, FSH, and gonadal hormone assays.

- Thyroid function tests (TSH and free T4) should be performed annually; treat primary hypothyroidism with levothyroxine after excluding cortisol deficiency.
- Evaluate adrenal function with early morning cortisol and ACTH; perform ACTH stimulation test if results are borderline to confirm adrenal insufficiency.
- Serum calcium, phosphorus, and PTH should be checked yearly to identify hypoparathyroidism; maintain calcium levels between 8–8.5 mg/dL to avoid hypercalciuria.
- Bone mineral density (BMD) assessment by DEXA scan is recommended every 2–3 years; a Z-score < –2 (below 50 years) or T-score < –2.5 (above 50 years) confirms osteoporosis.
- Ensure adequate calcium (up to 1300 mg/day) and vitamin D (1000 IU/day) supplementation from 9 years of age to maintain bone health.
- Optimization of transfusion regimen, iron chelation therapy, and nutritional support is essential before or alongside any hormonal replacement therapy.
- Close collaboration between hematologists, endocrinologists, and pediatricians is crucial for comprehensive endocrine management and to enhance growth, fertility, and quality of life in thalassemia patients.

REFERENCES

1. Toumba M, Sergis A, Kanaris C, et al. Endocrine complications in patients with Thalassaemia Major. Pediatr Endocrinol Rev. 2007;5(2):642-8.
2. Pantelakis S. Growth patterns in patients with thalassaemia major. Acta Paediatr Suppl. 1994;406:109-10.
3. Delvecchio M, Cavallo L. Growth and endocrine function in thalassemia major in childhood and adolescence. J Endocrinol Invest. 2010;33(1):61-8.
4. Rodda CP. Body proportions in patients with homozygous beta-thalassaemia. Acta Paediatr Suppl. 1994;406:107-8.
5. De Sanctis V, Soliman AT, Yassin MA, et al. Hypogonadism in male thalassemia major patients: pathophysiology, diagnosis and treatment. Acta Biomed. 2018;89(2-S):6-15.
6. Singha A, Mukhopadhyay P, Ghosh S. Thalidomide-Induced Primary Amenorrhea in a Patient WithHbE/Beta-Thalassemia, JCEM Case Rep. 2023;1(3):luad057.
7. Farmaki K, Tzoumari I, Pappa C, et al. Normalisation of total body iron load with very intensive combined chelation reverses cardiac and endocrine complications of thalassaemia major. Br J Haematol. 2010;148(3):466-75.
8. Srisukh S, Ongphiphadhanakul B, Bunnag P. Hypogonadism in thalassemia major patients. J Clin Transl Endocrinol. 2016;5:42-45.
9. Noetzli LJ, Panigrahy A, Mittelman SD, et al. Pituitary iron and volume predict hypogonadism in transfusional iron overload. Am J Hematol. 2012;87(2):167-71
10. Alexander EC, Faruqi D, Farquhar R, et al. Gonadotropins for pubertal induction in males with hypogonadotropic hypogonadism: systematic review and meta-analysis. Eur J Endocrinol. 2024;190(1):S1-S11.
11. Elsedfy HH, El Kholy M, Hamza RT, et al. Adrenal function in thalassemia major adolescents. Pediatr Endocrinol Rev. 2011;8 Suppl 2:295-9.
12. Huang KE, Mittelman SD, Coates TD, et al. A significant proportion of thalassemia major patients have adrenal insufficiency detectable on provocative testing. J Pediatr Hematol Oncol. 2015;37(1):54-9.
13. Uçar A, Öner N, Özek G, et al. Evaluation of the glucocorticoid, mineralocorticoid, and adrenal androgen secretion dynamics in a large cohort of patients aged 6-18 years with transfusion-dependent β-thalassemia major, with an emphasis on the impact of cardiac iron load. Endocrine. 2016;53(1):240-8.
14. Bornstein SR, Allolio B, Arlt W, et al. Diagnosis and Treatment of Primary Adrenal Insufficiency: An Endocrine Society Clinical Practice Guideline. J Clin Endocrinol Metab. 2016;101(2):364-89.

15. Soliman AT, Al Yafei F, Al-Naimi L, et al. Longitudinal study on thyroid function in patients with thalassemia major: High incidence of central hypothyroidism by 18 years. Indian J Endocrinol Metab. 2013;17(6):1090-5.
16. Pirinccioglu AG, Deniz T, Gokalp D, et al. Assessment of thyroid function in children aged 1-13 years with beta-thalassemia major. Iran J Pediatr. 2011;21(1):77-82.
17. Rombos Y, Tzanetea R, Konstantopoulous K. Chelation therapy in patients with thalassemia using the orally active iron chelators deferiprone. Hematol. 2000;85:115-7.
18. De Sanctis V, Soliman AT, Canatan D, et al. An ICET-A survey on Hypoparathyroidism in Patients with Thalassaemia Major and Intermedia: A preliminary report. Acta Biomed. 2018;88(4):435-44.
19. De Sanctis V, Soliman AT, Elsefdy H, et al. Bone disease in β thalassemia patients: past, present and future perspectives. Metabolism. 2018;80: 66-79.
20. Vogiatzi MG, Autio KA, Schneider R, et al. Low bone mass in prepubertal children with thalassemia major: insights into the pathogenesis of low bone mass in thalassemia. J Pediatr Endocrinol Metab. 2004;17(10):1415-21.
21. Marcon A, Motta I, Taher AT, et al. Clinical Complications and Their Management. Hematol Oncol Clin North Am. 2018;32(2):223-36.
22. Incorvaia C, Parmeggiani F, Mingrone G, et al. Prevalence of retinopathy in diabetic thalassemic patients. J Pediatr Endocrinol Metab. 1998;11 Suppl 3:879-83.

15

CHAPTER

Imaging in Thalassemia

Sukrita Bhattacharjee

INTRODUCTION

Thalassemia patients require frequent monitoring of various parameters to assess the effects of frequent blood transfusions, ineffective erythropoiesis, iron overload and related complications. Imaging plays a critical role in this, especially in detecting complications related to iron overload, organ damage, and other long-term effects of the disease and its treatments. The focus on imaging in thalassemia management is on assessing key organs that are prone to damage due to the disease's chronic nature and frequent blood transfusions.

ASSESSMENT OF IRON OVERLOAD[1-4]

MRI for cardiac iron (T2 MRI)* **(*Table 1*)**:

- *Indication*: Cardiac iron overload is one of the most serious complications of thalassemia, which leads to heart failure and arrhythmias. *MRI T2** is used to assess the level of iron accumulation in the myocardium.
- T2* MRI monitoring for cardiac iron overload should start based on ferritin levels and transfusion history
- *Serum ferritin is not a direct predictor of myocardial iron overload,* so T2 MRI should not be delayed until ferritin is very high.

TABLE 1: Cardiac MRI T2* thresholds indicating severity of myocardial iron overload with corresponding management strategies and suggested monitoring intervals.

T2* value (ms)	Cardiac iron overload severity	Clinical interpretation and management recommendation	Recommendations for monitoring
>20 ms	Normal	No significant myocardial iron overload. Routine monitoring	Repeat every 2 years
10–20 ms	Mild to moderate overload	Increased risk of cardiac dysfunction. Optimize chelation	Repeat annually
<10 ms	Severe overload	High risk of cardiotoxicity. Intensive chelation (combination therapy)	Repeat every 6 months
<6 ms	Critical overload	Very high risk of heart failure and arrhythmias. Close cardiac monitoring and aggressive iron chelation mandatory	

- *Even patients with ferritin < 1,000 ng/mL may develop cardiac iron overload,* especially in poorly chelated cases.
- Attain baseline T2* MRI value for cardiac iron at age 8 years

Interpretation

Liver iron concentration (MRI T2* or R2* imaging):[1,2]

- *Indication*: The liver is a major site of iron deposition in thalassemia patients and MRI can be used to evaluate liver iron concentration:
  - Start monitoring at age 8 years
  - Serum ferritin > 800 ng/mL
  - *Frequency*: Every 2 years if normal, annually in mild to moderate iron overload, and 6 monthly in severe overload

Interpretation[5,6]

Refer to **Table 2**.

CARDIAC IMAGING

Echocardiography[1,2,7-10]

- Diastolic dysfunction (early sign) **(Table 3)**
- Impaired LV relaxation is common even before systolic dysfunction.
- *Systolic dysfunction (late manifestation)*:
  - Reduced LV ejection fraction (LVEF < 50% is significant).
  - Subclinical systolic dysfunction may occur even with preserved LVEF
  - Strain imaging [global longitudinal strain, (GLS)] is more sensitive.
- *Right heart changes*:
  - RV dysfunction secondary to pulmonary hypertension
  - TR velocity >2.8 m/s suggests pulmonary pressure elevation.
- *Pulmonary artery hypertension*:[1,2,11]
  - More common in NTDT patients
  - Key echocardiographic parameters and cutoffs for assessment are summarized in **Table 4**.

TABLE 2: Liver T2* (ms), R2* (Hz), and LIC thresholds for grading hepatic iron overload, with corresponding severity classification and recommended chelation management strategies.

Liver T2* (ms)	R2* (Hz) range	LIC equivalent (mg Fe/g dry weight)	Severity of iron Overload	Management recommendations
>6.3	<88	<3 mg Fe/g	Normal	Routine monitoring
2.8–6.3	88–263	3–7 mg Fe/g	Mild to moderate	Optimize chelation therapy
1.4–2.7	263–555	7–15 mg Fe/g	Severe	Intensify chelation (consider combination therapy)
<1.4	>555	>15 mg Fe/g	Critical	High risk of liver fibrosis/cirrhosis, requires urgent intervention

TABLE 3: Echo-based grading of left ventricular diastolic dysfunction with corresponding Doppler and hemodynamic features.

Grade	Echo findings
Grade 1: Impaired relaxation (normal LAP)	↓ E-wave, ↑ A-wave, E/A ratio < 0.8, normal E/e', normal LA volume
Grade 2: Pseudo normal (elevated LAP)	E/A ratio 0.8–2.0, ↑ E/e' (>14), ↑ LA volume (>34 mL/m²), mild pulmonary hypertension
Grade 3: Restrictive filling (severely elevated LAP)	E/A ≥ 2.0, E/e' >14, markedly ↑ LA volume, ↑ pulmonary pressures

(E-wave: early filling; A-wave: atrial contraction; e' velocity: early diastolic mitral annular velocity; LA: left atrium; LAP: left atrial pressure)

   - PASP= 4 × (TR velocity) ^{2} + right atrial pressure (assumed or measured).
   - If TR velocity approaches or exceeds 3.0 m/s, or if symptoms like dyspnea, syncope occur → refer for right heart catheterization (gold standard for PAH diagnosis).
- *Other common findings*:
   - *Left atrial enlargement* (due to chronically high filling pressures)
   - *Mild mitral/tricuspid regurgitation*
   - *Pericardial effusion* (rare, late stage)

Speckle Tracking Echocardiography[12]

- *Reduced global longitudinal strain (GLS)*: Decreased LV-GLS in β-thalassemia major patients compared to healthy controls, suggests subclinical systolic dysfunction.
- *Right ventricular (RV) and atrial strain*: Reduced RV-GLS and altered atrial strain parameters, indicate early involvement.
- *Correlation with iron overload*: certain studies have found associations between reduced strain values and myocardial iron overload, emphasizing speckle tracking echocardiography's (STE's) potential in early detection.

Clinical Implications

- *Early detection*: STE can identify myocardial dysfunction before changes are evident in conventional echocardiography, allowing for timely intervention.
- *Monitoring tool*: Regular STE assessments can aid in monitoring cardiac function over time, especially in patients undergoing chelation therapy.
- *Risk stratification*: Incorporating STE findings can enhance risk assessment and guide therapeutic decisions in β-thalassemia major management.

Recommended Monitoring Protocol

Refer to **Table 5**.

Echo Red Flags in Thalassemia

- LVEF drop below 55% repeat ECHO every 3–6 months
- E/e' > 14
- Progressive LA enlargement
- Worsening GLS (≤18% abnormal)
- RV dysfunction or ↑ PASP
- Appearance of new regurgitant lesions

Cardiac MRI (For Detailed Structural and Functional Assessment)

IF echocardiography raises concerns.

BONE HEALTH IMAGING

- *Dual-energy X-ray absorptiometry (DEXA) scan:*[13-16]
   - *Indication*: Thalassemia patients are at high risk of osteoporosis due to anemia, iron overload, and the side effects of chelation therapy (especially

TABLE 4: Key echocardiographic parameters and cutoffs for assessment of pulmonary hypertension.

Echo parameter	Interpretation	Key cutoff
Tricuspid regurgitation (TR) Jet velocity	Estimate pulmonary artery systolic pressure (PASP)	>2.8 m/s suspicious for PAH
Right ventricular (RV) size and function	RV dilation, hypokinesia if advanced	
Right atrial (RA) enlargement	Suggests chronically elevated right-sided pressures	
Interventricular septal flattening	Seen in systole if pressure overload is significant	
Pulmonary acceleration time (PAT)	Shortened (<100 ms) if pulmonary pressures high	

deferoxamine, which can affect bone metabolism).

- *Interpretation*: DEXA measures bone mineral density (BMD) to assess for osteoporosis or osteopenia, common in adult thalassemia patients. It also plays a role in guiding therapy for the same. T-score is used to measure BMD by comparing a patient's BMD to that of a healthy 30-year-old adult of same sex.

When to Start Therapy Based on DEXA Results (Table 6)

- Start monitoring at age 10 years
- *Follow-up*: Every *12 months* to assess response in case of bisphosphonates.
- *Follow-up*: Every *6–12 months* to monitor bone density when using Denosumab.

In children and adolescents (up to 20 years old), *Z-scores* are used *(NOT T-scores)* to assess bone health because their bones are still growing and mineralizing. The *Z-score* compares a child's bone mineral density (BMD) to what is expected for their *age, sex, and size.*[15,16] Z score interpretation is summarized in **Table 7**.

Osteoporosis cannot be diagnosed on a low Z-score alone. It requires:

- A Z-score ≤-2.0
- A clinically significant fracture history, such as:
    - ≥ 2 long bone fractures before age 10 years, or
    - ≥3 long bone fractures before age 19 years, or
    - Vertebral compression fracture(s).

Adjustments needed: In children who are *short for age* or *have delayed growth*, BMD must be adjusted for *height age or bone age*. Otherwise, DEXA may falsely suggest low BMD.

TABLE 5: Recommended echocardiographic monitoring schedule for early detection of cardiac dysfunction.

Parameter	Frequency	Comments
Baseline echocardiography	Start at age 10 years (earlier if indicated)	Full LV/RV function + diastolic assessment
Routine 2D echo	Annually	Earlier if symptomatic or iron overload
Tissue Doppler imaging (TDI)	Annually	Essential for early dysfunction
Speckle tracking/strain echo	Every 1–2 years if available	Detects early systolic dysfunction
TR velocity and PASP	Annually	Screen for pulmonary hypertension
After high Ferritin or cardiac T2 MRI worsening	Repeat echo in 6 months	To assess for evolving dysfunction

TABLE 6: DEXA T-score categories for bone health status with corresponding management recommendations.

DEXA T-score	Bone health status	Recommended intervention
>–1.0	Normal bone mineral density (BMD)	No specific treatment, monitor every 1–2 years
–1.0 to –2.5	Osteopenia	Calcium, vitamin D, physical activity; monitor every 1 year
≤ –2.5	Osteoporosis	Bisphosphonates (1st line) or RANK ligand inhibitors
≤–2.5 with fractures	Severe osteoporosis	Bisphosphonates ± Denosumab (RANK ligand inhibitor)

Always interpret Z-scores along with:
- Growth measurements
- Pubertal stage
- Nutrition
- Disease status (like thalassemia and chronic illnesses)
- History of fractures

Currently, Indian data on use of DEXA scan in pediatric population is scanty.

- *X-ray Imaging of bone deformities*[13-17] ***(Table 8)***:
  - *Indication*: X-rays are used to monitor skeletal deformities, can also detect extramedullary hematopoiesis (EMH)

ABDOMINAL IMAGING

- *Ultrasound:*[17] Abdominal ultrasound can be used:
  - To assess the spleen's size and function.
  - To detect gallbladder stones, hepatic size and echotexture

TABLE 7: Bone mineral density Z-score interpretation, outlining thresholds for normal, borderline, and low bone density with corresponding clinical implications.

Z-score range	Interpretation	Clinical meaning
≥ –1.0	Normal	Bone density appropriate for age and sex
Between –1.0 and –2.0	Low bone density for age (borderline)	May require close monitoring, especially if risk factors present
≤ –2.0	Low bone density for chronological age	Suggests significantly lower than expected BMD for age; evaluate underlying causes

TABLE 8: Radiographic features of bone changes in chronic anemia, with key appearances, sites, and clinical significance.

Feature	X-ray appearance	Affected regions	Clinical significance
Osteopenia/ osteoporosis	Generalized bone demineralization, cortical thinning	Spine, hips, knees, hands, ankles	High fracture risk
Epiphyseal widening	Delayed skeletal maturation, widened growth plates	Long bones, wrists, knees, ankles	Growth disturbances
Subchondral Bone resorption	Irregular joint margins, subchondral cysts	Hip, knee, ankle	Early osteoarthritis
Osteoarthritis	Joint space narrowing, osteophytes	Hips, knees, shoulders	Progressive joint degeneration
Vertebral changes	Biconcave ("fish-mouth") vertebrae, platyspondyly	Thoracic and lumbar spine	Risk of compression fractures
Sclerosis and joint deformity	Patchy increased density, joint erosions	Knees, ankles, hands	Advanced joint damage
Pes planus (Flatfoot)	Collapsed arch, talar flattening	Ankle, foot	Weakening of foot structure
Skull changes (hair-on-end appearance)	Vertical striations due to expanded diploic space	Skull (frontal and parietal bones)	Marrow expansion, seen in severe anemia
Facial bone deformities (Rodent Facies)	Prominent maxilla, widened zygomatic bones	Skull, facial bones	Thalassemic facies from marrow expansion
Subperiosteal new bone formation	Periosteal reaction along long bones	Long bones, skull	Bone stress response to marrow hyperplasia

- To detect the presence of any thrombus, especially in case of NTDT by using Doppler ultrasonography
  - Recommended frequency: Annually (every 6 months if values are abnormal)
- *FibroScan (transient elastography)*: Noninvasive imaging technique widely used to assess liver stiffness, which correlates with liver fibrosis.[18,19] Interpretation is summarized in **Table 9**.
  - Baseline assessment around age 5–10 years
  - Monitoring for transfusion-dependent patients-requiring repeated transfusions, on iron chelation: Every 1–2 years
  - More frequent assessments (every 6–12 months) for those at higher risk:
    - Serum ferritin > 1,000 ng/mL. or hepatic MRI T2* showing signs of iron overload
    - Persistently elevated ferritin levels despite iron chelation or suspicion of inadequate chelation
    - increased risk of cirrhosis (chronic hepatitis B or C infection, evidence of increasing liver stiffness)
  - Pretransplant evaluations

TABLE 9: Correlation of liver stiffness measurements (kPa) with METAVIR fibrosis stages, outlining interpretation from minimal fibrosis to cirrhosis.

Liver stiffness measurement (kPa)	Fibrosis stage (METAVIR)	Interpretation
0–5.1	F0–F1	Minimal to no fibrosis
>7.9	F2	Significant fibrosis
10.3	F3	Severe fibrosis
11.9	F4	Cirrhosis

- *MRI or CT scanning (in certain cases)*:
  - *Indication*: MRI or CT scans may be used for more detailed splenic imaging if there is suspicion of complications, such as splenic infarction or rupture.

BRAIN IMAGING[20]

- MRI is used to assess the size and morphology of the pituitary gland, which can be damaged by iron overload
- MRI/CT brain can also detect the presence of any thrombus.

Extramedullary Hematopoiesis (EMH) Surveillance[1,2,21-23]

Extramedullary hematopoiesis (EMH) can cause mass effect symptoms, including spinal cord compression, respiratory distress, and organ dysfunction. Imaging is essential for diagnosis, treatment planning, and monitoring response to therapy. Imaging for detection of EMH is necessary for NTDT patients at the slightest clinical suspicion.

Imaging for EMH—Diagnosis and Baseline Assessment

Refer to **Table 10**.

CONCLUSION

Imaging plays a pivotal role in the comprehensive management of thalassemia, providing essential insights into the extent of iron overload, organ dysfunction, and treatment response. Regular and systematic use of imaging modalities such as cardiac and hepatic MRI, echocardiography, DEXA scans, and ultrasound enables early detection of complications, guiding timely therapeutic adjustments and improving long-term outcomes. MRI-based iron

TABLE 10: Imaging modalities for diagnosing extramedullary hematopoiesis (EMH), highlighting clinical indications, characteristic findings, and preferred applications by site.

Imaging modality	Clinical indication	Key findings	Preferred for
X-ray (spine and chest)	Initial detection of paraspinal or rib expansion EMH	Paraspinal soft tissue shadows, rib expansion	Simple screening tool
Ultrasound (USG)	Screening for hepatic/ splenic EMH	Hyperechoic or mixed echogenic lesions	Liver, spleen
MRI (T1/T2-weighted, with contrast if needed)	First-line for paraspinal EMH	Lobulated soft tissue mass, isointense on T1, hyperintense on T2	Spinal EMH (assessing cord compression)
CT scan (with contrast)	Evaluates thoracic, retroperitoneal, and pelvic EMH	Well-defined, nonenhancing soft tissue masses	Chest, abdomen, pelvis involvement
PET-CT (if malignancy suspected)	Differentiates EMH from tumors	Metabolically inactive soft tissue masses (vs. malignancies which are FDG-avid)	Atypical cases, suspicion of malignancy

quantification remains the gold standard for assessing myocardial and hepatic iron, while echocardiographic techniques—including tissue Doppler and strain imaging—facilitate early recognition of subclinical cardiac dysfunction. Bone densitometry and skeletal imaging are critical for monitoring osteopathy, a frequent comorbidity in these patients. Ultimately, an integrated, multidisciplinary imaging approach ensures proactive monitoring, personalized chelation strategies, and better quality of life for individuals living with thalassemia.

SUMMARY OF IMAGING RECOMMENDATIONS

- Start monitoring by imaging from 8 years of age for iron overload and 10 years for cardiac and bone health
- MRI imaging should not be delayed for ferritin levels to exceed >1,000 ng/mL (TDT) in case of cardiac MRI T2*
- *Annual imaging*: MRI (cardiac and liver), echocardiogram, and DEXA scan. Ultrasound, and follow-up imaging for organ complications.
- *As clinically indicated*: MRI of the brain or pituitary gland, bone X-rays for deformities, and more advanced imaging like CT scans for the spleen or organs with potential complications.
- Pulmonary artery hypertension and extramedullary hematopoiesis are more common in NTDT patients. Should be detected promptly for early intervention.

Imaging Recommendations for Thalassemia Management

Refer to **Table 11**.

TABLE 11: Recommended imaging modalities in thalassemia and iron overload disorders, detailing clinical indications, monitoring frequency, target organs, and key clinical considerations for ongoing management.

Imaging modality	Clinical indication	Frequency	Target organ/ system	Clinical considerations
MRI T2*/R2* for liver iron concentration	Quantification of hepatic iron overload	Every 2 years if normal, annually in mild to moderate iron overload and 6 monthly in severe overload	Liver	Gold standard for non-invasive liver iron assessment; guides chelation therapy adjustments
MRI T2* (cardiac iron)	Detection of myocardial iron overload *TDT*: After age 10 years *NTDT*: Ferritin >800/mL		Heart	Essential for pre-venting iron-induced cardiomyopathy; values <20 ms indicate risk
Echocardiography (ECHO)	Evaluation of cardiac function	Annually (more frequent if cardiac dysfunction suspected)	Heart	Assesses ventricular function, pulmonary hypertension, and heart failure risk
DEXA scan	Screening for osteoporosis and bone deformities	Annually, starting at age 10 years	Skeletal system	Important in patients with growth retardation, fractures, or suspected osteopenia
Abdominal ultrasound	Evaluation of hepa-tosplenomegaly, and gallstones	Annually	Liver and spleen	Identifies splenic enlargement, liver fibrosis, and biliary complications

REFERENCES

1. Cappellini MD, Farmakis D, Porter J, et al. Guidelines for the Management of Transfusion-Dependent Thalassaemia, 4th ed. Nicosia (CY): Thalassaemia International Federation; 2021.
2. Taher A, Musallam K, Cappellini MD, et al. Guidelines for the Management of Non-Transfusion-Dependent Thalassaemia (NTDT), 2nd ed. Nicosia (CY): Thalassaemia International Federation; 2017.
3. Ministry of Health and Family Welfare, Government of India. Guidelines for Prevention and Control of Hemoglobinopathies in India. New Delhi: National Health Mission; 2016.
4. Wood JC. Magnetic resonance imaging measurement of iron overload. Hematology Am Soc HematolEduc Program. 2011;2011(1): 443-50.
5. Pipaliya N, Patel M, Patel K, et al. Comparison of tissue elastography with magnetic resonance imaging T2* and serum ferritin quantification in detecting liver iron overload in patients with thalassemia major. Clin Gastroenterol Hepatol. 2017;15(2):292–8.e1.
6. Krittayaphong R, Viprakasit V, Saiviroonporn P, et al. Myocardial iron overload assessment by T2* magnetic resonance imaging in adult transfusion-

dependent patients with acquired anemias. J Magn Reson Imaging. 2012;35(1):134-9.

7. Pennell DJ, Udelson JE, Arai AE, et al. Cardiovascular function and treatment in β-thalassemia major: a consensus statement from the American Heart Association. Circulation. 2013;128(3):281-308.
8. Karamanou AG, Hamodraka ES, Vrakas SC, et al. Assessment of left ventricular and atrial diastolic function using two-dimensional strain imaging in patients with β-thalassemia major. Eur J Haematol. 2014;92(1):59-65.
9. Sadeghpour A, Kiavar M, Alizadehasl A, et al. Echocardiographic findings in thalassemia major: a case report and literature review. J Cardiovasc Thorac Res. 2012;4(2):57-9.
10. Nagueh SF, Smiseth OA, Appleton CP, et al. Recommendations for the evaluation of left ventricular diastolic function by echocardiography: an update from the American Society of Echocardiography and the European Association of Cardiovascular Imaging. Eur Heart J Cardiovasc Imaging. 2016;17(12):1321-60.
11. Derchi G, Forni GL, Formisano F, et al. Pulmonary hypertension in well-transfused thalassemia major patients. Blood Cells Mol Dis. 2014;52(4):189-93.
12. Patsourakos D, Aggeli C, Dimitroglou Y, et al. Speckle tracking echocardiography and β-thalassemia major. A systematic review. Ann Hematol. 2024;103:3335-56.
13. Vogiatzi MG, Macklin EA, Fung EB, et al. Prevalence of fractures among the thalassemia syndromes in North America. Bone. 2006;38(4):571-5.
14. Giusti A, Pinto V, Forni GL. Management of osteoporosis in adult thalassemia patients. Mediterr J Hematol Infect Dis. 2014;6(1):e2014063.
15. Dede AD, Trovas G, Chronopoulos E, et al. Bone disease in β-thalassemia major and intermedia: a review of pathophysiology, diagnosis, and treatment. J Musculoskelet Neuronal Interact. 2016;16(1):30-42.
16. Krueger D, Tanner SB, Szalat A, et al. DXA reporting updates: 2023 official positions of the International Society for Clinical Densitometry. J Clin Densitom. 2024;27(1):101437.
17. Bachrach LK, Gordon CM; Section on Endocrinology. Bone densitometry in children and adolescents. Pediatrics. 2016;138(4):e20162398.
18. Perifanis V, Vlachaki E, Sinakos E, et al. Transient elastography may predict liver iron overload in adult thalassemia patients. Blood. 2008;112(11):5407.
19. Cassinerio E, Fraquelli M, Volpato E, Ret al. Liver fibrosis in adult thalassemia patients assessed by transient elastography. Blood. 2007;110(11): 3820.
20. Noetzli LJ, Panigrahy A, Hyderi A, et al. Pituitary iron and volume predict hypothalamic-pituitary axis dysfunction in transfusional iron overload. J Clin Endocrinol Metab. 2012;97(8):E1893-9.
21. Wang Z, Zhou X, Zhou W, et al. MRI characteristics of paraspinal extramedullary hematopoiesis in beta-thalassemia: a study of 26 cases. Eur J Radiol. 2019;116:18-24.
22. Bernaudin F, Vernant JP, Begue P, et al. Paraspinal extramedullary hematopoiesis in Cooley's anemia: successful treatment by low-dose irradiation. Br J Haematol. 1998;103(1):191-3.
23. Taher AT, Musallam KM, Cappellini MD. Thalassemia intermedia: an update. Mediterr J Hematol Infect Dis. 2009;1(1):e2009004.

16

CHAPTER

Hematopoietic Stem Cell Transplant for Thalassemia Major

Vikram Mathews

INTRODUCTION

Need for HSCT in thalassemia major: For patients with beta thalassemia major, an allogeneic hematopoietic stem cell transplant (HSCT) is still the only accessible and effective treatment option. Due to wider availability of this curative therapy, its use is growing quickly in India and other developing nations. The main idea is that hematopoietic stem cells (HSC) can be transferred from a donor to a recipient, giving the recipient a new donor-derived hematopoietic system. Clinical outcomes for people with this condition following such a procedure have steadily improved due to significant advancements over the past 20 years. Nowadays, it is feasible to expect a favorable transplant outcome of more than 90% in patients with good risk characteristics.[1] Success rates are getting close to 80%, even for patients with high-risk characteristics. Better risk-stratified conditioning programs and more efficient supporting care have been used to achieve these gains.[1,2] Building capacity and expanding the number of facilities that can provide this treatment are necessary because thalassemia is a major public health issue in the nation.

PRETRANSPLANT RISK ASSESSMENT AND STRATIFICATION OF PATIENTS WITH THALASSEMIA MAJOR

Using liver size (>2 cm), liver fibrosis, and insufficient iron chelation, patients with beta thalassemia major receiving myeloablative allogeneic (SCT) are categorized into three risk groups (Pesaro Class I, II, and III).[3,4] Patients are categorized as Class I if they have none of the aforementioned risk factors, Class II if they have one or two of these risk factors, and Class III if they have all three of the negative risk factors (summarized in **Table 1**). Class I and II patients are thought to be low risk and have good long-term results after allogeneic stem cell transplantation.[3,4] Class III patients, on the other hand, are considered high risk and have inferior outcomes following an SCT. However, in a population with poor medical treatment before SCT, the above risk stratification is limited by its failure to recognize[2] the significant heterogeneity among patients in Class III. The Pesaro risk stratification[3,4] does not recognize a very high risk subset of Class III in these populations, perhaps because

TABLE 1: Risk factors and risk groups on pretransplant evaluation of patients with thalassemia major undergoing an HSCT.

Risk factors	Risk groups

• Liver size (>2 cm)
• Presence of liver fibrosis
• Inadequate iron chelation
	• Class I—none of the risk factors present
	• Class II—at least one risk factor but not all
	• Class III—all 3 risk factors present
	  ○ Class III low risk—class III without either liver size > 5 cm below costal margin or age > 7 years
	  ○ Class III high risk—class III with both liver size > 5 cm below costal margin and age > 7 years

such patients hardly exist in Western nations. Given the growing availability of allo-SCT in many developing nations with sizable patient populations, it is critical to identify this high-risk population in order to appropriately adjust SCT protocols.[2,5,6] Additionally, it must be stressed that SCT is contraindicated in patients who already have evidence of severe end-organ damage from high iron overload leading to organ dysfunction, such as cardiac failure or cirrhosis; such patients, even if considered for SCT should only be done in centers with substantial experience and expertise with handling these issues.

IMPORTANCE OF DOING HSCT AT A YOUNG AGE AND PREFERABLY BEFORE THE AGE OF 7 YEARS

In a 2007 review of a large data set from India, retrospective analysis of characteristics influencing clinical outcome helped uncover a very high-risk subset of a conventional Class III group (Class III high risk) that included patients aged ≥7 years and having a liver size ≥5 cm prior to transplant.[2] An international collaborative investigation conducted in 2010 further confirmed the detrimental effects of age (≥7 years) and liver size (> 2 cm).[7] The fact that these two groups' SCT results differed even though they received the same protocols highlights the importance of this distinction. Class III and more specifically Class III high risk (Class III HR)[8] subset have a high risk of graft rejection and regimen-related toxicity (RRT), especially sinusoidal obstruction syndrome (SOS), leading to multi-organ failure and death. These complications are perhaps related to the high degree of alloimmunization and iron overload-related end-organ damage in this cohort. Even in sophisticated nations that have experience with transplanting such populations, the rejection rate can reach 34%.[9]

SOURCE OF STEM CELLS AND ALTERNATIVE STEM CELL DONORS FOR HSCT IN THALASSEMIA MAJOR

Although the frequency of both acute and chronic GVHD is minimal in this primarily pediatric group, bone marrow (BM) has been the preferred source of stem cells in nonmalignant hematological illnesses to lower the risk of GVHD.[10,11] When employed, peripheral blood stem cell transplants (PBSC) have been linked to quicker engraftment and a decreased need for blood product support during the post-transplant phase[12-14] and have additionally been lead to a decreased rate of graft rejection.[11]

The best stem cell donor is an HLA-identical sibling donor. Unfortunately, only about a third of patients with thalassemia major have an HLA-matched sibling donor, which limits access to an SCT for these patients. There is a rare possibility of another related donor, such as a parent, grandparent, or cousin, being HLA identical, though the prior probability of this is extremely low. In communities with a high incidence of consanguinity, the probability of a non-sibling related family donor being HLA-identical is higher.

Matched Unrelated Donors

Patients without a matched related donor may choose to use a matched unrelated donor (MUD) SCT. Prior to the development of high-resolution HLA typing, the early outcomes of this method were dreadful, with a 55% graft rejection rate.[15] Since then, MUD SCT has significantly improved, and high-resolution molecular HLA typing has become the norm for MUD selection. The results of MUD-treated malignant diseases are now on par with those of HLA-matched sibling transplants. According to recent data, the results of a completely matched (high-resolution typing) MUD SCT for thalassemia major are similar to those of a matched related donor; the only drawback is the higher expense of obtaining a matched unrelated donor product.[16] The outcome with mismatched MUD remains poor with a standard conditioning regimen and GVHD prophylaxis regimen and should preferably be avoided. The overall data would suggest that MUD SCT should only be considered in centers that have reasonable experience with this approach, high-resolution HLA typing with a full (10 of 10) match is the preferred donor, and in addition, they should ideally not have HLA-DP1 mismatches in the direction favoring graft rejection.[17]

Cord Blood Transplants

Over the past 10 years, the most rapidly expanding source of stem cells for allogeneic stem cell transplantation has been cord blood transfusions. There is, however, little information available for patients with thalassemia major. Two groups must be taken into consideration when using cord blood stem cells for allogeneic SCT in thalassemia major, as they differ significantly in terms of clinical outcome:

- *Related cord blood transplant*: When stem cells are obtained from a sibling who is either HLA-matched or partially mismatched
- *Unrelated cord blood transplant*: When an unrelated cord blood product is obtained from a cord blood bank as part of a donor search for an allogeneic SCT. Different levels of HLA mismatch may exist.

Using related cord blood, the Eurocord Transplant Group reported a 2-year probability of thalassemia-free survival of 79% in 33 patients with thalassemia.

For patients with thalassemia major, an unrelated cord blood transplantation actually expands the pool of possible donors. Regretfully, there isn't much data available. Nineteen cases were documented in a recent evaluation of six studies.[18] The cumulative graft failure rate was an alarming 52%, according to a 2011 research by Ruggeri et al. that combined data from three independent registries.[19] As of right now, an unrelated cord blood transplantation cannot be suggested outside of a research trial.

Even for a related fully matched donor cord blood, one would prefer to defer the transplant till the is about 2 years and use a conventional bone marrow or a peripheral blood stem cell graft from the same donor, which is likely to be associated with faster engraftment, lower treatment-related mortality and improved survival.

Haplo-identical Stem Cell Transplants

Over the past few years, haplo-identical stem cell transplants have attracted a lot of attention worldwide. Even in the absence of graft T cell depletion, novel conditioning and GVHD prophylactic regimens have shown markedly improved clinical outcomes. The TFS was almost 67% and the graft rejection rate was 27% in one small study ($n = 22$) utilizing T cell depletion grafts. Recently, there have been some encouraging studies about the use of grafts with CD3αβ T cell depletion.[20] The use of pretransplant immunosuppression, followed by GVHD prophylaxis with post-transplant cyclophosphamide (PTCy), has been associated with a significant improvement in survival, with one report demonstrating a 3-year event-free survival of 96%.[21,22] This is an option for patients in India, but should be preferably done with considerable available expertise and support systems to monitor and treat various viral reactivations as well as other infective, GVHD and long-term morbidity issues that are relatively more common with a haplo-identical SCT.

TRANSPLANT PROCEDURE

Before initiating the procedure, a detailed pre-transplant evaluation of the patient and the donor is done to confirm diagnosis, HLA match status, and also to exclude any condition that is a contraindication to proceeding with a transplant, in both the recipient and the donor. The conventional conditioning regimen that is used is a combination of busulfan and cyclophosphamide. More recently, several novel conditioning regimens have been introduced, and a popular alternative is a treosulfan-based conditioning regimen that replaces busulfan and is better tolerated with fewer adverse events. Bernado et al. published the first report on the use of treosulfan as part of the conditioning regimen for thalassemia in a small series of 20 patients, 18 of whom had matched unrelated stem cell transplants and 45% of whom were Class III.[23] Due to its low hepatic and other toxicity profile across a broad range of AUCs, which eliminates the need for drug dose monitoring and makes it an appealing agent to use, the treosulfan-based conditioning regimen is well suited for patients with thalassemia major, including very high-risk patients.

Post-transplant patients need to be monitored carefully for engraftment. Patients continue to remain at high risk for infections for the first year. Additional complications that can occur in a proportion of cases and can occasionally be fatal include graft rejection and graft versus host disease, neither of which can be accurately predicted.

After transplantation, the iron overload status still needs to be treated. Phlebotomy is the recommended technique for removing iron after a successful transplant, as long as the patient is stable and hemoglobin level is more than 100 g/L. A volume of 6 mL/kg can be eliminated in a single sitting, and it can be repeated once every 14 days. The patient should begin chelation therapy if the hemoglobin level is insufficient or if phlebotomy is not feasible. It should be continued until the ferritin level is less than 100 ng/mL, which may take years. The optimal pharmacological agent(s) and chelation regimen post-transplant remain to be defined. In addition to chelation, these patients need close attention to immunization, endocrine and organ dysfunction secondary to iron overload.

CONCLUSION

Hematopoietic stem cell transplantation has revolutionized the management of β-thalassemia major, providing a potentially permanent cure for patients otherwise dependent on lifelong transfusion and chelation. Successful outcomes depend on timely referral, careful pretransplant risk assessment, optimal donor selection, and individualized conditioning protocols. Early transplantation, ideally before the age of 7 years and prior to the development of significant iron overload, offers the best prognosis. Matched sibling donor transplants remain the gold standard, while matched unrelated and haplo-identical transplants are expanding the curative possibilities in resource-limited settings. Advances in supportive care, novel conditioning regimens such as treosulfan-based protocols, and improved post-transplant monitoring have further enhanced survival and quality of life. As the capacity for HSCT expands in developing nations, integrating this curative modality into national thalassemia control programs can substantially reduce disease burden and transform patient outcomes for generations to come.

SUMMARY

1. Hematopoietic stem cell transplant (SCT) in thalassemia major remains the only widely available one-time curative treatment for this condition.
2. It is important to recognize risk features in these patients and consider alternative conditioning regimens and improved supportive care pre- and post-transplant.
3. It is important to reinforce the need to do an SCT where possible at a young age and preferably before the age of 7 years.
4. Matched sibling/related (MSD/MRD), matched unrelated (MUD) and even a haplo-identical donor are all options for these patients. MUD and haploidentical SCTs should be preferably done in a high-volume center with the availability of appropriate supportive infrastructure.

REFERENCES

1. Mathews V, Srivastava A, Chandy M. Allogeneic stem cell transplantation for Thalassemia major. Hematol Oncol Clin North Am. 2014;28(6):1187-200.
2. Mathews V, George B, Deotare U, et al. A new stratification strategy that identifies a subset of class III patients with an adverse prognosis among children with beta thalassemia major undergoing a matched related allogeneic stem cell transplantation. Biol Blood Marrow Transplant. 2007;13(8):889-94.
3. Lucarelli G, Galimberti M, Polchi P, et al., Bone marrow transplantation in patients with thalassemia. N Engl J Med. 1990;322(7):417-21.
4. Lucarelli G, Galimberti M, Polchi P, et al. Bone marrow transplantation in adult thalassemia. Blood. 1992;80(6):1603-7.
5. Hongeng S, Pakakasama S, Chuansumrit A, et al. Outcomes of transplantation with related- and unrelated-donor stem cells in children with severe thalassemia. Biol Blood Marrow Transplant. 2006;12(6):683-7.
6. Fang JP, Xu LH. Hematopoietic stem cell transplantation for children with thalassemia major in China. Pediatr Blood Cancer. 2010;55(6): 1062-5.
7. Sabloff M, Chandy M, Wang Z, et al. HLA-matched sibling bone marrow transplantation for beta-thalassemia major. Blood. 2010;117(5):1745-50.
8. Phrommintikul A, Sukonthasarn A, Kanjanavanit R, et al. Splenectomy: a strong risk factor for pulmonary hypertension in patients with thalassaemia. Heart. 2006;92(10):1467-72.
9. Chiesa R, Cappelli B, Crocchiolo R, et al., Unpredictability of intravenous busulfan pharmacokinetics in children undergoing hematopoietic stem cell transplantation for advanced beta thalassemia: limited toxicity with a dose-adjustment policy. Biol Blood Marrow Transplant. 2010;16(5):622-8.
10. Chandy M, Balasubramanian P, Ramachandran SV, et al. Randomized trial of two different conditioning regimens for bone marrow transplantation in thalassemia—the role of busulfan pharmacokinetics in determining outcome. Bone Marrow Transplant. 2005;36(10):839-45.
11. Rajasekar R, Mathews V, Lakshmi KM, et al. Cellular immune reconstitution and its impact on clinical outcome in children with beta thalassemia major undergoing a matched related myeloablative allogeneic bone marrow transplant. Biol Blood Marrow Transplant. 2009;15(5):597-609.
12. Mathews V, George B, Viswabandya A, et al. Improved Clinical Outcomes of High Risk beta Thalassemia Major Patients Undergoing a HLA Matched Related Allogeneic Stem Cell Transplant with a Treosulfan Based Conditioning Regimen and Peripheral Blood Stem Cell Grafts. PLoS One. 2013;8(4):e61637.
13. Iravani M, Tavakoli E, Babaie MH, et al. Comparison of peripheral blood stem cell transplant with bone marrow transplant in class 3 thalassemic patients. Exp Clin Transplant. 2010;8(1):66-73.
14. Ghavamzadeh A, Iravani M, Ashouri A, et al. Peripheral blood versus bone marrow as a source of hematopoietic stem cells for allogeneic

transplantation in children with class I and II beta thalassemia major. Biol Blood Marrow Transplant. 2008;14(3):301-8.
15. Gaziev D, Galimberti M, Lucarelli G, et al. Bone marrow transplantation from alternative donors for thalassemia: HLA-phenotypically identical relative and HLA-nonidentical sibling or parent transplants. Bone Marrow Transplant. 2000;25(8):815-21.
16. La Nasa G, Giardini C, Argiolu F, et al. Unrelated donor bone marrow transplantation for thalassemia: the effect of extended haplotypes. Blood. 2002;99(12):4350-6.
17. Fleischhauer K, Locatelli F, Zecca M, et al. Graft rejection after unrelated donor hematopoietic stem cell transplantation for thalassemia is associated with nonpermissive HLA-DPB1 disparity in host-versus-graft direction. Blood. 2006;107(7):2984-92.
18. Pinto FO, Roberts I. Cord blood stem cell transplantation for haemoglobinopathies. Br J Haematol. 2008;141(3):309-24.
19. Ruggeri A, Eapen M, Scaravadou A, et al., Umbilical cord blood transplantation for children with thalassemia and sickle cell disease. Biol Blood Marrow Transplant. 2011;17(9):1375-82.
20. Bertaina A, Merli P, Rutella S, et al. HLA-haplo-identical stem cell transplantation after removal of alphabeta+ T and B-cells in children with non-malignant disorders. Blood. 2014;124(5):822-6.
21. Wang F, Qu Y, Jiang H, et al. Allogeneic hemato-poietic stem cell transplantation for thalassemia major using matched unrelated donors and haploidentical related donors. Chin Med J (Engl). 2025;138(4):490-2.
22. Anurathapan U, Hongeng S, Pakakasama S, et al. Hematopoietic Stem Cell Transplantation for Severe Thalassemia Patients from Haploidentical Donors Using a Novel Conditioning Regimen. Biol Blood Marrow Transplant. 2020;26(6):1106-12.
23. Bernardo ME, Zecca M, Piras E, et al. Treosulfan-based conditioning regimen for allogeneic haematopoietic stem cell transplantation in patients with thalassaemia major. Br J Haematol. 2008;143(4):548-51.

17

CHAPTER

Psychological Support to Patients and Parents

Ved P Choudhry

INTRODUCTION

Thalassemia is an inherited genetic disorder and thus requires lifelong treatment. Thalassemia is a chronic disease presenting in the first year of life. The growth and development of thalassemia children primarily depends on how patients and family have learned to live with thalassemia.[1] In the early stages, these children are dependent on parents and family members and as they grow they must learn to take care of themselves.[2] The pediatrician along with the institution provides the initial treatment and all possible support and later the hematologist or physician provides the healthcare. In India, it has been observed that pediatricians continue to provide thalassemia care even during adulthood.

NEED FOR PSYCHOSOCIAL SUPPORT

There is no National Thalassemia Registry and therefore, there is no data on the burden of thalassemia and related disorders in our country. It is expected that there are nearly 1, 50,000 thalassemia major in India and similar no of patients with thalassemia intermedia, thalassemia sickle cell anemia, E beta-thalassemia disease, and thalassemia with other hemoglobinopathies are in India. Long-term survival along with good quality of life in these patients primarily depends upon the education and financial level of the parents and most importantly psychological and emotional support available to the patients and their family members throughout their life. There is lack of published data and randomized controlled trials to evaluate the impact of psychological support interventions in patients with thalassemia. However, the behavior and psychological problems along with multiple difficulties for regular blood transfusions to maintain the hemoglobin levels and adherence to iron chelation therapy have been observed in these children which plays a significant role in long term survival's and quality of life. In this section a detailed review of psychological problems in these children along with the possible interventions which will help them to improve the long term survivals and quality of life has been included.

The World Health Organization has defined health as a state of complete physical, mental and social wellbeing and not merely the absence of the disease.[3] Therefore, it is mandatory for healthcare professionals to also focus on clinical welfare including emotional and social issues besides treating the underlying diseases or disabilities. Hematologist/physician/pediatrician while treating thalassemia children should include siblings and parents for counseling, psychological and social issues.[4,5] Psychological problems requiring interventions at various stages of thalassemia care and control will be reviewed.

TIME OF DIAGNOSIS

Moment the parents learn that their child has thalassemia major which requires lifelong repeated blood transfusions, chelation therapy, and continuous monitoring and both parents are thalassemia minors. They go into a state of shock, phase of denial, anger, and guilt. They usually argue with their doctors that they have never heard of this disease and as they are perfectly normal. They refuse to accept that they are having any genetic problems. Many times they go to other doctors or institutions for the second opinion and confirmation of the diagnosis. The family generally needs maximum psychological support at this time. Family needs to be informed that (a) thalassemia carrier rate is as high as 17% in certain communities; (b) they should be educated regarding the genetics of the disease after confirming their diagnosis; (c) risks of subsequent children having thalassemia should be explained; (d) need for thalassemia carrier detection in the siblings and first family relationship should be explained; (e) family should get their child registered in the nearby thalassemia day care center; (f) parents should meet other thalassemia children and their parents at the day care center who are best to provide them psychological support and assurance that their child will do well with the current treatment; (g) need for regular transfusions and to maintain the pretransfusion hemoglobin at 10 g/dL; (h) parents should be counseled regarding the various support groups: (i) they should understand the need to become member of a thalassemia society and to co-operate with the society in their own interest. They need to be educated regarding various programs such as:

- Thalassemia has been included as a disability as per Rights of Persons with Disability (RPwD) act 2016.
- Need to get a Unique Disability Identity Card (UDID) and its benefits.
- Prime Minister Relief Fund for cure of thalassemia.
- *Rashtriya Arogya Nidhi* Scheme, *Ayushmaan Bharat* Scheme, income tax rebate, fare concessions for thalassemia patients
- Chief Minister Relief Fund
- State Specific Programs
- Some states give financial aid to all thalassemia patients.
- Corporate Social Responsibility (CSR) initiatives under which they support for the thalassemia screening programs, for Bone Marrow Transplant, chelation therapy, etc.
- Nongovernment organizations which provide support to these children in multiple ways.

Good counseling along with psychological support provides assurance and confidence to the family that they can continue the treatment of their child with the support of their doctor, day care center and thalassemia society. Thalassemics Societies provide all possible help to facilitate the parents to initiate therapy besides helping them to get support from various agencies. Thalassemia care providers should ensure (a) to provide necessary information to parents several times for their comprehension; (b) clear all concerns of the parents; (c) make arrangements to meet children with thalassemia for social support and developing confidence; (d) to provide psychological support, and (e) to help them to get aid from various government agencies.

INITIATION OF BLOOD TRANSFUSION

Parents are concerned about the pain for venous access, transfusion and its side effects. Families need to explain the technique through visual aids, pictures or showing them actual procedures on older children. Visiting a day care center where children are getting transfusions helps them to build confidence and trust. Family should be counseled about the frequency of blood, amount of blood transfusion during each visit and duration of transfusion, importance of maintaining Hb at 10 g/dL, its complications along with preventive measures and treatment of complications. Importance of leukoreduced blood transfusion and its cost should be explained.[6] During the initial blood transfusions, children are scared of the room and the surroundings, nurses, doctors, and they look to their parents for signals on how to react toward this novel situation, anxiety, etc. In a meta-analyses study on psychological interventions for needle related procedure, initiation of blood transfusion in children and adolescents distraction was found to be the most effective measure. In another study, bubble blowing during the procedure was found to reduce anxiety. Children at a later age may ask more questions about transfusion, frequent monitoring, invasive procedures such as MRI, ultrasound, FibroScan, etc., which need to be explained. All efforts should be made to answer the questions of children and parents by use of visual aids, books, pictures, videos, group discussions, etc. Information regarding genetics of thalassemia, need for cascade screening to determine the thalassemia status in the siblings and extended family members should be undertaken for the control of thalassemia. Families need to be counseled accordingly and the team should ensure all family members follow their advice. Family should be counseled regarding hematopoietic stem cell transplant (HSCT) which offers complete cure. Their doubts should be resolved and all possible information regarding the centers, the cost HSCT, and cure rates should be explained. Parents should be encouraged for HSCT and possible ways to collect funds from various sources. Parents should understand that HSCT results are best below 7 years of age and after 12 years the results are poorer. Please refer to the section on HSCT for further details.

INITIATION OF CHELATION

Parents should be informed regarding all the available chelating agents. They should be given support and guidance to tell them which chelator is best for their child and is associated with less side effects, distress, easy to administer and provides better quality of life.[7] Parents should be encouraged to develop a routine which is practical for them to administer chelator regularly and need to adhere to a schedule. Family should be explained that maintaining serum ferritin below 1,000 ng/mL is of utmost importance to avoid any damage to vital organs (heart, liver, and endocrine glands). Regular monitoring and use of incentives to the child are helpful for the adherence to therapy. Incentives may include verbal praise, stickers, toys, gifts, awards, etc., for cooperating with daily chelation. Children often struggle with adherence to chelation therapy and to maintain their serum ferritin levels.[8]

ADOLESCENCE

During adolescence adherence to medical treatment usually declines as the responsibility shifts from parents to adolescence before the child is fully matured and they take decisions which are driven by their emotions and their discussions with fellow thalassemics and friends. Parents with the help of a medical team can overcome these issues. Children during this time are concerned about their body images, short stature, pubertal development which cause psychological problems. Hemolytic facies if present now becomes their major concern which affects them as they are either getting inadequate attention or adverse reaction from classmates and opposite sex. Timely intervention by psychiatrists as well as enhancing their self-image and esteem, sense of humor, confidence, smartness, etc., helps them greatly. Encourage the children to get appropriate guidance for medical issues such as short stature and other medical problems. Psychologist support during this period is of great help to them.

TRANSITION TO ADULT CARE

Adherence to blood transfusions, chelation therapy and other treatments is lowest because of insufficient psychological support, new environment and adult medical providers which happens suddenly to which children are not prepared and are unable to adjust. They are shifting from their comfort zone and missing the play room in children thalassemia day care and company of their old friends with whom they have strong bonds and friendship for years. Discussion with these children for their care under the adult team should be discussed with them and they need appropriate counseling, support and assurance. This process should be gradual to help these children to cope with the new environment, stress etc. Good psychological support helps to convince these children to continue their treatment under adult care.

ADULTHOOD

During this period they are concerned about higher education, skill development, employment, and business opportunities. Most of the children's education is affected and their performance is poorer as compared with normal children as they are irregular in their school/college as they have to attend the day care center for transfusion and to their doctors for medical needs. However there are many who have excelled and have become professionals and entrepreneurs. These children require psychological support and guidance for their career in the area of their interest. Thalassemics Societies, doctors and psychologists expose them repeatedly to successful stories. All possible intervention related to their privileges for higher education and job opportunities should be imparted to the children and their parents. Information regarding RPWD act 2016 should be given to them. Parents who have their own business, involved in agriculture or any other type of jobs should encourage their children to join them.

MARRIAGE COUNSELING

All thalassemics should be explained again regarding the genetics of thalassemia and their doubts should be addressed to their satisfaction. They should be encouraged to develop relationships and plan for a successful married life.[9] Details of genetics, antenatal diagnosis and centers with these facilities should be provided.[10] It should be emphasized that they should not hide information that their child is having thalassemia major for the successful marriage life. Married life becomes difficult and chances of divorce are higher if such information is withheld. It is well known that in the Indian scenario to get the match is difficult when the other family learns about the life of persons with thalassemia. Intervention by psychologists, doctors, and thalassemia societies can be of great help in alleviating the concerns in this regard. It has been observed that few thalassemia major children have married together as they understand well the need of each other and they provide support to each other for transfusion and all other necessary treatment. They understand well that either they will adapt children to become parents or use in vitro fertilization facilities with donor sperm to have their children. Please refer to the section on control of thalassemia for further details.

DURING LIFE

Thalassemics are at higher risk of having growth disorders such as short stature, bone diseases such as osteopenia, osteoporosis due to poor maintenance of hemoglobin and iron overload. Iron overload can also cause cardiac and liver failure. These individuals need to be counseled and monitored to ensure that they maintain adequate levels of hemoglobin and serum ferritin levels. These persons can develop hepatitis B or C through blood and need monitoring for the same. Hepatitis B can be prevented by hepatitis B vaccination at diagnosis and subsequently booster dose every 5 years. Psychological support throughout their life plays an important role for the prevention, early diagnosis and institution of appropriate therapy.[11,12] These persons are at higher risk of developing various endocrine disorders. If they develop any endocrine disorders due to iron overload they need psychological support to explain to them the underlying reasons for its development and need for regular replacement therapy for the rest of their life. For detailed information on endocrine issues refer to the section on endocrine disorders. Persons with thalassemia have the same risk of having diseases as normal persons such as hypertension, pulmonary diseases, coronary diseases, etc. Persons with thalassemia continue to have multiple health challenges. Continuous and coordinated psychological, social, medical support goes a long way to help them to live near normal.

CONCLUSION

Thalassemia is an inherited genetic disorder requiring lifelong treatment with continuous monitoring for early detection and treatment of complications of the disease and its treatment. Medical treatment has significantly improved over the years resulting in near normal life. However, these children, parents and family members have multiple social, psychological and emotional problems which greatly affect the quality of life of these children. Parents' problems start the day the diagnosis of thalassemia is made on their loved ones. Parents undergo a state of shock, denial and guilt requiring maximum psychological support. Medical teams need to provide full details of genetics along with assurance to provide them regular transfusions, chelation therapy, necessary monitoring along with all possible support to ensure that their child will be looked after in all aspects. Visit to day care centers, interactions with other thalassemic children and assurance of total support from thalassemia society goes a long way to build the confidence of the family. They require psychological support throughout their life as they face new problems such as at school, adolescence, their shifting to the adult day care center, growth and developmental issues, higher education, carrier selection, etc., and during adulthood as they have to cope with the treatment of thalassemia in addition to challenges of their job, family life etc. Psychological support has to be individualized as everyone has different problems of their education, family, career, marriage etc. With continuous psychological support along with comprehensive current medical treatment and support from NGO, and Government support has significantly improved the long term survivals and quality of life of thalassemia children all over the World.

SUMMARY

- *Introduction*: Thalassemia is a lifelong inherited disorder; patient growth and quality of life depend on family understanding and continuous psychological support.

- *Need for support*: India has approximately 150,000 cases; emotional, social, and financial support are vital for survival and better outcomes.
- *At diagnosis*: Parents face denial and guilt; need counseling on genetics, carrier screening, disability benefits, and government support.
- *Blood transfusion*: Explain procedure, benefits, and risks using visual aids; reduce child anxiety through distraction.
- *Chelation therapy*: Educate on drugs, adherence, ferritin < 1000 ng/mL, and use incentives to encourage compliance.
- *Adolescence*: Address emotional and body image issues; ensure counseling for self-confidence and adherence.
- *Adult care transition*: Provide gradual shift and reassurance to maintain treatment continuity.
- *Adulthood*: Guide on education, jobs, and rights under RPwD Act to build independence.
- *Marriage counseling*: Teach genetic risks and antenatal testing; encourage openness with partners.
- *Life-long care*: Continued medical and psychological support prevents complications and improves quality of life.

REFERENCES

1. Seyedifar M, Dorkoosh FA ,Haemideh AA, et al. Health related quality of life and health utility values in beta thalassemia major patients receiving different types of iron chelator in Iran. Int J Hematol Oncol Stem Cell Research. 3016;10;224-31
2. Soni S, Thawani R, Idhate T, et al. Health related quality of life in patients with transfusion dependent thalassemia. Ind Pediatr. 2016;53;741-2.
3. World Health Organization. Constitution of the World Health Organization. [online] Available from https//www.who.int/about/governance/constitution [Last accessed October, 2025].
4. Lal A. Assessment and treatment of pain in thalassemia. Ann N Y Acad Sc. 2016;1368;65-72.
5. Manimala MR, Blount RL, Cohen LL. The effects of parental reassurance versus distraction on child distress and coping during immunisation. Children Health Care 2000;29;161-77.
6. Jaaniste, Hayes B, von Baeyer CL, et al. Providing children with information about forthcoming medical procedures and review and synthesis. Clin Psychol Sci Pract. 2000;14;124-43.
7. De Sanctus V, Solman AT, Elsedfy H, et al. Growth and endocrine disorders in thalassemia: the international network on endocrine complications in thalassemia (I-CET) position statement and guidelines. Ind J Endocrinal Metab. 2013;17;8-18.
8. Porter JB, Evangeli M, El-Beshlawy A. Challenges of adherence and performance with iron chelation therapy. Int J Hematol. 2011;94:453-60.
9. Yamashita R, Haines D, Mednick L, et al. Psychological support. In: Capelini MD, Farman's D, Porter J, Taher (Eds). Guidelines for management of transfusion dependent thalassemia (TDT), 4th edition. Cyprus: Thalassemia International Federation; 2021. pp. 244-65.
10. Thakur S, Singh S. Genetic counselling to prevent thalassemia & hemoglobinopathies in the Indian population. Perinatology. 2019;20;61-6.
11. Tanm HS, Oz F. Thalassemia major and associated psychological problems. A narrative review. Iran J Public Health. 2022;51;12-8.
12. Madani Meghna, Arora JS. Psychosocial Councelling. In: Manglani M, Radhakrishnan N, Dewan P, Chandra J (eds). Evidence-based IAP-PHI Guidelines for the Diagnosis and Management of Thalassemia-2023, 1st edition. New Delhi: Pediatric Hematology Oncology Chapter of the Indian Academy of Pediatrics; 2023.

18

CHAPTER

Recent Advances in Thalassemia Management

Mukul Aggarwal, Manoranjan Mahapatra

INTRODUCTION

For decades now, regular packed RBC transfusion with chelation and hematopoietic stem cell transplant (HSCT) has been established as the standard of care for patients with thalassemia. However, patients face problems related to access to regular and safe transfusions, alloimmunization, transfusion-related reactions, frequent hospital visits, school/work absenteeism, high iron overload despite chelation, frequently observed compliance issues, etc. With new progress in the point-of-care diagnosis of thalassemia, monitoring with FibroScan, approval of luspatercept for adult thalassemic, and availability of gene therapy in the US and Europe, the field of thalassemia management is undergoing rapid transformation. Several drugs that alter RBC and/or iron metabolism are in early clinical trials; some will become part of thalassemia care in the future. These advances are being discussed in this chapter. Further refining in HSCT techniques and care is beyond the scope of this and is being discussed elsewhere.

EMERGING ROLE OF COMPREHENSIVE CARE

As the patients of thalassemia major achieve a better quality of healthcare, their survival is improving, and so many comorbidities associated with the illness and aging are being recognized. These include complications related to the heart, liver, endocrine system, and other body organs. All of these required a team of specialists, involving their treating hematologist or physician, cardiologist, endocrinologist, hepatologist, transfusion services, nursing care, nutritionist, etc. The concept of a comprehensive thalassemia care clinic is emerging in this regard, where all these services are provided under one umbrella.

MODALITIES FOR IRON OVERLOAD

FibroScan

FibroScan is a noninvasive imaging technique used to assess liver stiffness, which can indicate fibrosis or cirrhosis. In thalassemia, FibroScan helps monitor liver health by providing a quick and painless way to evaluate the extent of liver fibrosis. This helps pick up advanced changes seen in advanced and prolonged hemosiderosis, as it is not sensitive to earlier alterations in liver histology.

Herbal products such as tea, curcumin, etc., are also being tried as natural chelators in formal trials.

NEW DRUGS IN THALASSEMIA (FIG. 1)

Luspatercept

Luspatercept is a recombinant fusion protein (modified extracellular domain of the human ActRIIB linked to human IgG1 fragment) that blocks transforming growth factor beta superfamily ligands, mainly activin B, growth differentiation factor 11 or BMPs and hence rebalances intracellular cell signaling, which favors late-phase erythroid maturation.

As per BELIEVE and BEYOND trials in transfusion-dependent and nontransfusion-dependent patients with thalassemia, respectively, it has shown improvement in transfusion burden and anemia with good tolerability.[1] Around 21.4% of patients had more than a 33% reduction, and around 7.5% had more than a 50% reduction in transfusion requirement in TDT, as compared to placebo. These responses were seen across all ages, regions, and transfusion burdens, but were more pronounced in non–β0/β0 patients and splenectomized patients.

While more than 50% had a rise of 1.5 g/dL in NTDT, with a low risk of thrombosis.[2,3] More than 75% of patients had a rise of at least 1 g/dL of Hb in the absence of transfusion, as compared to nil in the placebo group at weeks 13–24. Luspatercept group patients had a reduced PRBC requirement, with mean decreases of 6.2 RBC units (SD 5.7) during weeks 97–144 and 6.4 RBC units (4.3) during weeks 145–192.[4]

The majority of patients are not transfusion-free and data on the impact on iron overload is evolving; the decrease or stabilization of liver iron concentration has been demonstrated starting week 96. Among the responding patients, meaningful improvements were seen in health-related quality of life and physical functions (TranQoL and SF-36 questionnaires).[5] Side effects include headache, diarrhea, extremity pain, backache, hypertension, extramedullary pseudotumor (10.4%), thrombosis (2.1%), hyperuricemia, with serious adverse events in up to 23% patients. Luspatercept is commercially available in India, and real-world experience is accumulating with mixed but expected results in patients. (unpublished data and personal communications).

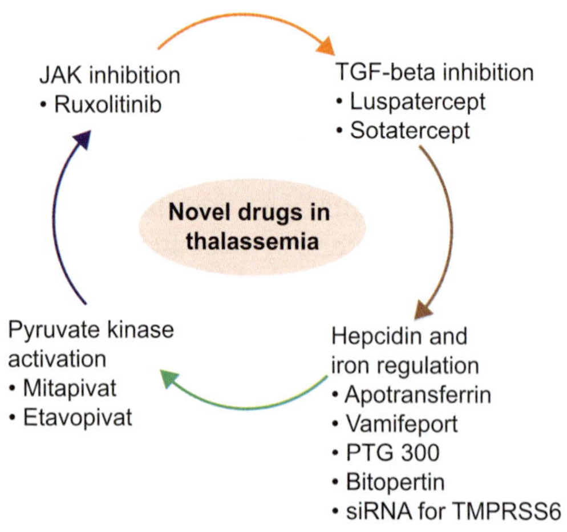

FIG 1: The novel drugs in thalassemia and their mechanism of action.

JAK Inhibitors

JAK inhibitors have been investigated in thalassemia for their potential to modulate ineffective erythropoiesis and reduce splenomegaly. Ruxolitinib, a JAK2 inhibitor, was tried at a dose of 10 mg BD in TDT patients. Trial results showed a decrease in spleen size, and an increase in hepcidin; however, no significant improvements were seen in pretransfusion hemoglobin or reduction in transfusion needs, and further trials were not started.[6]

Mitapivat

Mitapivat is an oral activator of pyruvate kinase, an enzyme involved in glycolysis—the crucial ATP-generating metabolic pathway in RBCs. In thalassemia, there is relative oxidative stress due to increased RBC turnover, and relative deficiency of NADH, hence, mitapivat is being studied for its potential to improve red blood cell function and reduce anemia by enhancing energy production in red blood cells. In a phase 2 study in NTDT, it provided a sustained rise of >1g/dL in Hb in 80% of patients and reduced markers of hemolysis as well as ineffective erythropoiesis.[7] Responses were better in alpha thalassemia. Common adverse events were insomnia (50%), dizziness (30%), headache (25%), and renal dysfunction. Phase 3 studies in both TDT (ENERGIZE-T) and NTDT (ENERGIZE) are underway.

Alteration in Iron Metabolism

Nontransferrin-bound or free iron can affect RBCs by decreasing their survival in blood and production in marrow. Alteration in iron metabolism has been proposed to improve anemia and decrease iron accumulation in thalassemia. The master regulator of iron is hepcidin, which acts via ferroportin at various levels.

Hepcidin mimetics (PTG 300),[8] an inhibitor of ferroportin (VIT 2763, vamifeport),[9] apotransferrin (upregulates hepcidin),[10] glycine transport inhibitor bitopertin[11] have shown above effects in animal models but failed in clinical studies. Rusfertide, a peptidic mimetic of hepcidin, prevents iron reaccumulation in the absence of phlebotomies in patients with hereditary hemochromatosis in a phase 2 study. This could hold promise in secondary hemochromatosis, as in thalassemia as well.[12] Similarly, the inactivation of TMPRSS6 with small interfering RNA (siRNA) or antisense oligonucleotides (ASO) in preclinical studies in mice led to increased hepcidin levels and improved IE.[13] Further clinical studies are underway. In a phase 2A trial in NTDT patients, Vamifeport showed improvement in hematological parameters, iron parameters, and biomarkers for erythropoietic activity, along with improvement in serum iron and transferrin saturation.[14]

IMMUNOMODULATORS IN THALASSEMIA

Although HbF induction with thalidomide has been discussed elsewhere in the book, it is important to consider this recent advancement, now commonly employed in both TDT and NTDT patients. Moderate reduction in transfusion requirement to complete independence has been documented in some patients, with responses varying from 25 to 70% across studies, depending on the study population. There is a danger of thrombotic complications and other side effects of thalidomide, which should be discussed before initiation of therapy, especially in females of reproductive age group.

THROMBOEMBOLISM IN TDT AND NTDT

Due to various reasons like erythroid microparticles, free heme and nitric oxide consumption and reactive oxygen species, thromboembolism is more prevalent in TDT and NTDT patients. There are more venous events in NTDT and more arterial events in TDT, which are increased after splenectomy. Thromboembolism has been described in up to 1.65% of thalassemia patients, with TDT patients 4.38 times less likely than NTDT patients to have thrombosis.[15] Preventive therapy with aspirin has been explored, especially in splenectomized patients, high nRBC counts ($>300 \times 10^6$/L), pulmonary hypertension, surgery and pregnancy.[16] Venous thrombosis is managed as per guidelines with heparin or direct oral anticoagulants for prolonged periods.[17]

GENE THERAPY

Gene therapy has been postulated as a one-time therapy for transfusion-dependent beta-thalassemia. It has been approved by the US FDA and EMA for use in adult and pediatric patients. G-CSF mobilizes the stem cells, transduced with BB 305 lentiviral vector, which codes for the beta-globin gene that is (βA-T87Q) Hb.[18] Another approach is to use autologous HCS modified at erythrocyte lineage-specific enhancer of the BCL11A gene (to reactivate hemoglobin F) using CRISPR/CAS9 or zinc-finger nuclease. The latter approach, termed Gene editing, is very promising but is still not approved.[19]

Ex vivo activation is undertaken under cytokines, stem cell factor, etc., as the patient undergoes busulfan-based myeloablative conditioning. As per the trial results, transfusion independence was achieved in almost 90% of the participants along with a reduction in ineffective erythropoiesis. Subsequently, 72% of the patients had decreased or discontinued their iron chelation therapy over time and had a reduction in side effects due to iron overload.[20] Gene therapies also resulted in the improvement of health-related quality of life scores in physical, psychological, social, and environmental domains.[21]

Potential side effects include myelotoxicity because of conditioning, mucositis, anorexia, neutropenic fever, sinusoidal obstruction syndrome of the liver, very high cost, and development of MDS/MDS, and cerebral adrenoleukodystrophy in some of the recipients. Advantages include one-time therapy, with no need for a suitable donor, and other transplant-associated complications like GVHD, hemorrhagic cystitis, etc.

There have been efforts to start gene therapy trials in India, with preclinical work in progress at several institutions. Cas9 RNP-ssODN-based nucleotide conversion at the HBG promoter with up to 57% of long-term engrafting human HSPCs in NBSGW mice has been tried by the CMC Vellore group, offering a promising gene therapy approach for thalassemia.[22] They also identified an 11-kb sequence, encompassing a putative repressor region (PRR) to β-globin exon-1 (βE1), as the core deletion that ablates HbA and exhibits superior HbF production. These edited hematopoietic stem and progenitor cells (HSPCs) could repopulate for long-term hematopoiesis in immunocompromised mice, producing HbF-positive cells in vivo. They suggest this gene editing could be a beneficial approach.[23]

CONCLUSION

Thalassemia management is rapidly evolving with newer drugs like luspatercept and mitapivat reducing transfusion needs, noninvasive tools improving monitoring, and gene therapy offering a potential cure. With multidisciplinary care and advancing therapies, patients can expect improved survival, quality of life, and future hope for definitive treatment.

SUMMARY

- New advances in diagnostics and therapeutics in thalassemia have the potential to revolutionize the lives of patients.
- FibroScan of the liver can substitute liver biopsy needed before transplant and become noninvasive means to assess hepatic hemosiderosis.
- Drugs like luspatercept and mitapivat reduce the transfusion burden in a good percentage of patients and help decrease iron overload.
- Iron metabolism can be altered to benefit patients by decreasing hemosiderosis, as has been shown in preclinical studies. Clinical trial data is awaited.
- Gene therapy is here and approved for TDT, although it is currently very expensive and long-term data is evolving.

REFERENCES

1. Cappellini MD, Viprakasit V, Taher AT, et al. A phase 3 trial of luspatercept in patients with transfusion-dependent beta thalassemia. N Engl J Med. 2020;382(13):1219-31.
2. Taher AT, Cappellini MD, Kattamis A, et al. Luspatercept for the treatment of anaemia in non-transfusion-dependent beta thalassaemia (BEYOND): a phase 2, randomised, double-blind, multicentre, placebo-controlled trial. Lancet Haematol. 2022;9(10):e733-44.
3. Hermine O, Cappellini MDD, Taher AT, et al. Effect of luspatercept on red blood cell (RBC) transfusion burden, iron chelation therapy (ICT), and iron overload in adults with transfusion-dependent β-thalassemia (TDT) from the BELIEVE trial: a long-term analysis. Blood. 2022;140(suppl 1):8215-7.
4. Cappellini MD, Viprakasit V, Georgiev P, et al. Long-term efficacy and safety of luspatercept for the treatment of anaemia in patients with transfusion-dependent β-thalassaemia (BELIEVE): final results from a phase 3 randomised trial. Lancet Haematol. 2025;12(3):e180-9.
5. Cappellini MD, Taher AT, Piga A, et al. Health-Related Quality of Life Outcomes for Patients with Transfusion Dependent Beta-Thalassemia Treated with Luspatercept in the Believe Trial. Blood. 2020;136:8-9
6. Taher AT, Karakas Z, Cassinerio E, et al. Efficacy and safety of ruxolitinib in regularly transfused patients with thalassemia: results from a phase 2a study. Blood. 2018;131(2):263-5.
7. Kuo KHM, Layton DM, Lal A, et al. Safety and efficacy of mitapivat, an oral pyruvate kinase activator, in adults with non transfusion dependent alpha-thalassaemia or beta-thalassaemia: an open-label, multicentre, phase 2 study. Lancet. 2022;400(10351):493-501.
8. Preza GC, Ruchala P, Pinon R, et al. Minihepcidins are rationally designed small peptides that mimic hepcidin activity in mice and may be useful for the treatment of iron overload. J Clin Invest. 2011;121(12):4880-8.
9. Taher A, Kourakli-Symeonidis A, Tantiworawit A, et al. Safety and preliminary pharmacodynamic effects of the ferroportin inhibitor vamifeport (VIT 2763) in patients with non-transfusion dependent beta thalassemia (NTDT): results from phase 2A study. HemaSphere. 2022;6:173-4.
10. Garbowski MW, Evans P, Vlachodimitropoulou E, et al. Residual erythropoiesis protects against myocardial hemosiderosis in transfusion-dependent thalassemia by lowering labile plasma iron via transient generation of apotransferrin. Haematologica. 2017;102(10):1640-9.
11. Taher AT, Viprakasit V, Cappellini MD, et al. Haematological effects of oral administration of bitopertin, a glycine transport inhibitor, in patients with non transfusion-dependent beta-thalassaemia. Br J Haematol. 2021;194(2):474-7.
12. Kowdley KV, Modi NB, Peltekian K, et al. Rusfertide for the treatment of iron overload in HFE-related haemochromatosis: an open-label, multicentre, proof-of-concept phase 2 trial. Lancet Gastroenterol Hepatol. 2023;8(12):1118-28.
13. Schmidt PJ, Toudjarska I, Sendamarai AK, et al. An RNAi therapeutic targeting Tmprss6 decreases iron overload in Hfe(-/-) mice and ameliorates anemia and iron overload in murine beta-thalassemia intermedia. Blood. 2013;121(7):1200-8.
14. Taher A, Kourakli-Symeonidis A, Tantiworawit A, et al. S272: safety and preliminary pharmacodynamic effects of the ferroportin inhibitor vamifeport (VIT-2763) in patients with non-transfusion-dependent beta thalassemia (NTDT): results from a phase 2A study. HemaSphere. 2022;6:173-4.
15. Taher A, Isma'eel H, Mehio G, et al. Prevalence of thromboembolic events among 8,860 patients with thalassaemia major and intermedia in the Mediterranean area and Iran. Thromb Haemost. 2006;96(4):488-91.
16. Saliba AN, Musallam KM, Taher AT. How I treat non-transfusion-dependent β-thalassemia. Blood. 2023;142(11):949-60.
17. Bou-Fakhredin R, Cappellini MD, Taher AT, et al. Hypercoagulability in hemoglobinopathies: Decoding the thrombotic threat. Am J Hematol. 2025;100(1):103-15.
18. Locatelli F, Thompson AA, Kwiatkowski JL, et al. Betibeglogene autotemcel gene therapy for non-β0/β0 genotype β-thalassemia. N Engl J Med. 2022;386:415-27.
19. Frangoul H, Altshuler D, Cappellini MD, et al. CRISPR-Cas9 gene editing for sickle cell disease and beta-thalassemia. N Engl J Med. 2021;384:252-60.
20. Thompson A, Locatelli F, Yannaki E, et al. Restoring iron homeostasis in pts who achieved

transfusion independence after treatment with betibeglogene autotemcel gene therapy: Results from up to 7 Years of follow-up. Paper presented at: Blood; 2021

21. Kwiatkowski JL, Locatelli F, Walters MC, et al. Improvement in health-related quality of life following treatment with betibeglogene autotemcel in patients with transfusion-dependent β- thalassemia enrolled in phase 3 studies. Blood. 2021;138:3085.
22. Chandraprabha PB, Azhagiri MKK, Venkatesan V, et al. Enhanced fetalhemoglobin production via dual-beneficial mutation editing of the HBG promoter in hematopoietic stem and progenitor cells for β-hemoglobinopathies. Stem Cell Res Ther. 2024;15(1):504.
23. Venkatesan V, Christopher AC, Rhiel M, et al. Editing the core region in HPFH deletions alters fetal and adult globin expression for treatment of β-hemoglobinopathies. Mol Ther Nucleic Acids. 2023;32:671-88.

19

CHAPTER

Role of NGO and Corporates for Control and Management of Thalassemia

JS Arora

INTRODUCTION

Thalassemia is an inherited lifetime crippling disorder requiring frequent repeated blood transfusions, risks of transfusion transmitted infections, disabilities, vital organ failure and premature deaths. It requires a multi-faceted approach involving prevention, early detection, treatment, and support services. Initially family stroll pillar to post in search of tagging it a wrong diagnosis or trying to cure with alternative miraculous methods. Many times, they fall prey to miracle healers resulting in severe consequences, including delaying or avoiding necessary medical treatment, potential financial exploitation, and even death.

While governmental efforts are crucial, the involvement of Non-Governmental Organizations (NGOs) and Corporates can greatly enhance the effectiveness of control and management strategies. NGOs and Corporates play pivotal roles in complementing governmental efforts by synergizing their resources, expertise, and networks, NGOs and Corporates can foster comprehensive approaches toward combating thalassemia and improving the quality of life for affected individuals.

KEY AREAS OF NON-GOVERNMENTAL ORGANIZATIONS

NGOs provide services in three key areas—psychological support, management, and control.

Psychological support is crucial and diverges at four stages of life in thalassemics so dealt separately.

At Diagnosis

Parents undergo a series of situations once their child is diagnosed with thalassemia—shock, denial, sadness, anger, and adaptation.

It is especially important to help parents accept and learn to effectively cope with their child's chronic medical condition at this early stage. One of their most important immediate concerns is getting reliable information, opportunities to ask questions and share concerns. Introducing the family to an appropriately experienced family with a child who has thalassemia can be a helpful learning experience for parents of young children while decreasing feelings of loneliness, helplessness and hopelessness.

During Childhood

Children with thalassemia frequently miss school for medical appointments and transfusions negatively impacting their education, NGOs need to educate the school about their child's condition and set-up plans to support the child when he needs to miss school.

Providing advanced information to older children about transfusions and other invasive medical procedures fosters trust, reduces uncertainty, eliminates misconceptions, enhances belief in their ability to cope with uncertainties and minimizes distress.

Adolescence

Thalassemic adolescents experience feelings of shame, stigmatization, uncertainty of future and fear of death. They are vulnerable to nonadherence to medical regimens. Psychological well-being impacts on adherence to chelation treatment and hence on survival. NGOs regularly interact with patients and caregivers and motivate for self-care and adherence. NGOs create social groups and use text messaging and mobile phone app as an alternative approach

Adult Care

Adulthood in thalassemic is more challenging. Increased blood requirement and hospital visits, moving out of hometown for higher education or job, relationship, family life and future uncertainties are grueling and need tough decisions. NGOs are always keen to support their health necessities, especially migration for education and employment. NGOs organize capacity building workshops and "adult thalassemic alone" meetings to give them an opportunity to deliberate on common issues and find solutions.

THE ROLE OF NGOS IN THALASSEMIA CONTROL AND MANAGEMENT

- *Awareness campaigns*: Organize educational workshops, seminars, and community outreach programs to disseminate information about thalassemia, its causes, symptoms, and prevention methods. Collaborate with healthcare professionals, schools, universities, and community leaders to reach a wider audience and dispel myths and misconceptions surrounding the disorder. Utilize various media platforms, including social media, television, radio, and print, to amplify awareness messages.
- *Screening programs*: Establish screening centers in collaboration with healthcare facilities to facilitate easy access to carrier screening and counseling services for individuals at risk of carrying thalassemia genes. Implement population-based screening initiatives targeting high-risk communities to identify carriers and provide them with appropriate information and support. Advocate for mandatory premarital and prenatal screening policies to reduce the transmission of thalassemia genes and prevent new cases from occurring.
- *Support services:* Provide access to healthcare resources, including medical treatment, medications, blood transfusions, and specialized care, through partnerships with hospitals, clinics, and healthcare providers. Establish support groups and online forums to facilitate peer support, information sharing, and networking among patients, caregivers, and healthcare professionals.
- *Blood donation drives:* Organize regular blood donation drives to ensure a steady supply of blood. Collaborate with local blood banks, hospitals, and community organizations to maximize the impact of blood donation initiatives.
- *Advocacy and policy:* Advocate for the rights of individuals with thalassemia, including access to affordable and quality healthcare, education, employment, and social inclusion. Lobby governments and policymakers to allocate resources for thalassemia prevention, treatment, and research, and to implement policies that prioritize the needs of affected individuals and families. Collaborate with international organizations, professional societies, and other stakeholders to promote global initiatives and standards for thalassemia care and management.

- *Capacity building:* Provide training and resources for healthcare professionals to enhance their knowledge and skills in diagnosing and managing Thalassemia effectively. Facilitate workshops and conferences to share best practices and promote collaboration among healthcare providers.
- *Research and innovation:* Support research initiatives aimed at developing new treatments and curative options for Thalassemia patients. Foster partnerships with academic institutions, research organizations, and pharmaceutical companies to accelerate progress in thalassemia research.

THE ROLE OF CORPORATES IN THALASSEMIA CONTROL AND MANAGEMENT

Corporates have the potential to make significant contributions to thalassemia control and management through corporate social responsibility (CSR) initiatives, philanthropic partnerships, and employee engagement programs.

- *Financial support:* Allocate funds toward thalassemia awareness campaigns, screening programs, treatment facilities, research projects, and support services through corporate donations, grants, and sponsorships. Establish corporate foundations or trusts dedicated to thalassemia prevention and care, with a focus on addressing the specific needs of affected communities and populations.
- *Employee engagement:* Encourage employee involvement in thalassemia-related volunteer activities, fundraising events, blood donation drives, and advocacy campaigns to raise awareness and support for the cause. Provide paid time off or incentives for employees participating in blood donation programs or volunteering with thalassemia support organizations, thereby fostering a culture of CSR and community engagement.
- *Partnerships and collaborations:* Forge partnerships with NGOs, healthcare institutions, government agencies, and other stakeholders to leverage collective resources, expertise, and networks for thalassemia control and management initiatives. Engage in public-private partnerships to develop sustainable and scalable solutions for thalassemia prevention, treatment, and support, with a focus on innovation, efficiency, and impact.
- *Advocacy and awareness:* Use corporate platforms, channels, and networks to raise awareness about thalassemia and promote healthy behaviors, preventive measures, and early detection strategies among employees, customers, suppliers, and the wider community. Advocate for supportive policies, legislation, and regulations at the corporate, national, and international levels to address thalassemia-related challenges and facilitate access to care and support services.

SYNERGIZING THE ROLE OF NGOS AND CORPORATES

Collaboration between NGOs and Corporates is essential for maximizing the impact of thalassemia control and management efforts. By synergizing their resources, expertise, and networks, NGOs and Corporates can develop comprehensive and sustainable solutions that address the multifaceted needs of individuals and communities affected by thalassemia.

- *Strategic partnerships:* Establish formal partnerships and collaborative frameworks between NGOs and Corporates to align goals, priorities, and activities related to thalassemia control and management. Jointly develop and implement projects, campaigns, and initiatives that leverage the strengths and resources of both sectors, ensuring synergy, efficiency, and impact.

- *Resource mobilization:* Pool financial, human, and technical resources from both NGOs and Corporates to support thalassemia-related programs, activities, and services, maximizing the utilization and effectiveness of available resources. Explore innovative funding mechanisms, such as social impact investing, corporate matching grants, and cause-related marketing, to generate sustainable funding streams for thalassemia initiatives.
- *Capacity building:* Share knowledge, skills, and best practices between NGOs and Corporates through training programs, workshops, and mentorship opportunities, enhancing the capacity of both sectors to address thalassemia-related challenges. Foster cross-sectoral learning and collaboration to promote innovation, creativity, and continuous improvement in thalassemia control and management strategies.

RECOMMENDATION

Non-Governmental Organizations

- *Awareness campaigns:* Conduct educational campaigns targeting schools, communities, and healthcare facilities to raise awareness about its prevention, and management. Utilize various channels such as social media, workshops, seminars, and information pamphlets to disseminate information.
- *Support services:* Provide psychosocial support to patients and their families, including counseling services and support groups. Offer financial assistance for medical expenses, treatment, and medication through fundraising efforts and partnerships with healthcare institutions.
- *Blood donation drives:* Organize regular blood donation drives to ensure a steady supply of blood. Collaborate with local blood banks, hospitals, and community organizations to maximize the impact of blood donation initiatives.
- *Advocacy and policy influence:* Advocate for policies that promote screening programs for thalassemia carriers, prenatal testing, and access to affordable treatment options. Lobby government bodies and healthcare authorities to prioritize thalassemia prevention and management in public health agendas.
- *Capacity building:* Provide training and resources for healthcare professionals to enhance their knowledge and skills in diagnosing and managing thalassemia effectively. Facilitate workshops and conferences to share best practices and promote collaboration among healthcare providers.
- *Research and innovation:* Support research initiatives aimed at developing new treatments and curative options for thalassemia patients. Foster partnerships with academic institutions, research organizations, and pharmaceutical companies to accelerate progress in thalassemia research.

Corporates

- *Financial support:* Allocate funds for thalassemia awareness campaigns, patient support programs, and research projects through CSR initiatives. Establish grant programs or donation matching schemes to encourage employee contributions toward thalassemia-related causes.
- *Employee engagement:* Organize employee volunteering activities such as blood donation camps, health screenings, and awareness sessions on thalassemia prevention and management. Offer flexible work policies to accommodate

employees who are thalassemia patients or caregivers, ensuring they have access to necessary healthcare services and support.

- *Partnerships and sponsorships:* Partner with NGOs, healthcare institutions, and government agencies to sponsor thalassemia awareness events, fundraisers, and educational programs. Sponsor research projects and clinical trials focused on thalassemia treatment and management, fostering collaboration between academia and industry.
- *Education and training:* Offer employee training sessions on thalassemia awareness, prevention strategies, and support resources, empowering staff to become advocates for the cause. Encourage corporate leaders and decision-makers to participate in thalassemia-related conferences, summits, and policy discussions to drive meaningful change at the organizational and societal levels.
- *Product innovation and accessibility:* Explore opportunities for product innovation, such as affordable diagnostic tools, medications, and medical devices tailored to the needs of thalassemia patients ensuring that costs do not hinder patient's access to life-saving interventions.

Live Examples

National Thalassemia Welfare Society (NTWS) intervention—New Thalassemia units in Delhi and NCR, free prenatal diagnostic facility at Lok Nayak Hospital Govt of Delhi. FREE all three chelating agents for patients registered in Delhi Government Hospitals. This has been adopted by many other states. Organized National Conferences, Symposiums, Workshops and Webinars to update doctors and educate thalassemia families. Instrumental in creating new thalassemia associations in various cities and disseminating information through National Thalassemia Bulletin.

NTWS played a key role in bringing thalassemia in the list of disabilities in the *"Disability Act 2016"*.

Providing treatment support in form of free checkup, investigations, medication and BMT support.

NTWS and Pahuja Trust for Blood Disorders funded research projects on Thalidomide with premier institutes.

CORPORATE SUPPORT

NTWS initiated a project on thalassemia free Delhi NCR with support of CSR funding.

Coal India Limited provide financial assistance up to ₹10 lakh for Bone Marrow Transplant Thalassemia Bal Sewa Yojana of Ministry of Health and Family Welfare.

CONCLUSION

Effective control and management of thalassemia require collaborative efforts involving NGOs, corporates, governments, healthcare providers, and communities. By adhering to the guidelines outlined above and adopting collaborative strategies, NGOs and corporates can make significant contributions to reducing the burden of thalassemia and improving the quality of life for individuals and families affected by this genetic disorder.

SUMMARY

- *Introduction*: Thalassemia is a lifelong genetic disorder needing frequent transfusions and chelation; NGOs and corporates can complement government efforts by providing prevention, treatment, and sustained patient support.
- *Psychological support*: NGOs assist families at diagnosis, during childhood, adolescence, and adulthood—helping cope with emotional distress, promoting

adherence to treatment, and facilitating education and social inclusion.
- *Awareness and screening*: NGOs run educational campaigns, community programs, and screening initiatives, advocating mandatory premarital/ prenatal screening to prevent new cases.
- *Support services and blood drives*: NGOs provide counseling, financial aid, treatment support, and organize regular blood donation drives in partnership with hospitals and blood banks.
- *Advocacy and capacity building*: NGOs influence public policy, train healthcare providers, and support research for better management and cure options.
- *Corporate contributions*: Through CSR, corporates offer financial support for awareness, treatment, and research; engage employees in volunteering, blood donation, and advocacy; and innovate affordable diagnostic and treatment solutions.
- *Collaborative strategies*: NGOs and corporates form strategic partnerships, pool resources, share expertise, and co-develop sustainable thalassemia prevention and care programs.
- *Impact examples*: NTWS initiatives include free chelating agents in Delhi, prenatal diagnostics, national conferences, policy advocacy, and research funding; Coal India funds up to ₹10 lakh for BMT under Bal Sewa Yojana—showing tangible benefits of NGO-corporate collaboration.

20

CHAPTER

Translational Research in Thalassemia

Manisha Madkaikar, Neha Kargutkar, Roshan Colah, BV Babu

INTRODUCTION

The thalassemia syndromes are among the most common human monogenic disorders worldwide, as well as in India. Chronicity of the disease and the high cost of life-long treatments result in a significant burden on the healthcare system. In spite of the knowledge generated through research over several decades, a lot needs to be achieved for more effective prevention programs and more successful and affordable therapeutic approaches.

RESEARCH FOR MORE EFFECTIVE PREVENTION PROGRAMS

Carrier detection and genetic counseling are pillars of the prevention of thalassemia. Premarital screening of young adults to prevent marriage between two carrier individuals and antenatal screening of pregnant women in the first trimester needs to be focused on reducing the birth of affected children.

- High quality uniformly collected epidemiological data from all states are needed on prevalence of carriers, molecular genotypes, number of patients requiring treatment, number of births and deaths of β thalassemia patients to maintain a national database to enable health planners and policy makers to translate this into early interventions for management and prevention in regions where they are most needed.[1]
- AI-based algorithms based on different CBC parameters are being developed to alert physicians to test for thalassemia. Simple mobile app-based applications with high sensitivity will definitely benefit the prevention programs.[2] However, they are still in the initial stages of development and need validation using large data sets and their ability to differentiate from iron deficiency, which is prevalent in India.
- Innovative approaches for encouraging premarital testing, addressing issues of social stigma and improving community acceptance of marriage counseling are required to prevent births with thalassemia.
- One of the important challenges faced by couples at risk is the limited availability of prenatal diagnostic (PND) facilities. Currently, approved techniques for fetal sampling are invasive and are available only in metropolitan cities, hence families has to travel long distances for PND, thereby reducing the acceptance. Translation of antenatal screening into prenatal testing of the fetus is still challenging for the prevention program. The establishment of more specialized centers for PND and implementation research to identify and address the gaps is important. Identification of 3 to 20% cell-free fetal DNA (cffDNA) in

maternal plasma has paved the way for noninvasive prenatal diagnosis (NIPD) for thalassemia. Different techniques like droplet digital PCR (ddPCR), next generation sequencing (NGS), etc., are being explored to detect fetal mutations in maternal blood accurately, which is critical for diagnosis.[3] Again, the technical complexities, limited validation and cost of testing are currently the challenges which, once overcome, can transform the prevention programs.

RESEARCH TO IMPROVE MANAGEMENT OF THALASSEMIAS

Transfusion and iron chelation therapy: In the last two decades, we have witnessed expansion in centers offering hematopoietic stem cell transplantation (HSCT) nationwide. However, most patients with thalassemia still continue on transfusion therapy.

- Till curative options for thalassemia become widely available, there is a need to optimize the transfusion practices for thalassemia patients and achieve optimum iron chelation to avoid complications due to iron overload.
- Antigen-matched blood transfusion practices for thalassemia patients are known to reduce the rate of alloimmunization. Implementation research to ensure accurate typing of thalassemia patients, creation of an antigen-matched donor database and creation of a system that will facilitate uninterrupted antigen-matched blood supply are required to improve the transfusion services for thalassemic patients in India.
- There is also a need for health systems research to assess and implement cost-effective strategies for providing safe blood units to prevent transfusion-transmitted diseases and their complications.[4]
- Optimum iron chelation is necessary in chronically transfused thalassemics to prevent long-term complications. Multiple challenges exist for the optimum use of iron chelation facilities, which include limitations of the assays for assessment of the iron burden and adequacy of iron chelation, variability in the pharmacokinetics of iron chelators, adverse effects to iron chelators affecting its use, acceptability, compliance and cost and access to iron chelation which need to be addressed through systematic research. In addition, implementation research is required to ensure the availability of these drugs and to promote drug adherence.[5]
- One of the important areas of research is understanding the regulation of γ globin gene expression and identifying safer therapeutic options for HbF induction, which can reduce transfusion requirements. Repurposing of several drugs especially those with ability to induceg-globinexpressionisbeingstudied for TDT. These include hydroxyurea, thalidomide and derivatives, short-chain fatty acids, erythropoietin and derivatives, and DNA methylation inhibitors (e.g., 5-azacytidine and decitabine), sirolimus, or their combinations, etc. These drugs have shown benefits in the management of thalassemia patients especially to reduce transfusion requirements.[6,7] However, further studies are required for their efficacy and long term safety.
- Raising hemoglobin levels using erythroid maturation agent like luspatercept and improving ineffective erythropoiesis by pyruvate kinase pathway activators like mitapivat have shown beneficial effects in early studies.[7]
- Allogeneic transplantation of hematopoietic stem cells (allo-HSCT) is the only currently available curative option. Unfortunately, upfront mortality in high-risk patients and the unavailability of the HLA-matched donor often restricts its universal application. Research in the area of making alternative donor

transplantation safer and efficacious using different conditioning regimens is an important area of research which may benefit not only thalassemia patients but many other diseases amenable to cure by allo-HSCT.[8]

- Gene therapy is a promising curative therapeutic option for thalassemia patients, especially for whom allo-HSCT is not possible. Research in increasing the efficiency and accuracy of gene editing using tools like CRISPR/Cas9, ZFN, TALENs, etc., and the delivery systems is required to improve the outcome after therapy.[9,10]

CONCLUSION

Overall, there is a need to plan studies to generate evidence relevant to our population, increase interdisciplinary coordination to generate new diagnostic or therapeutic options for better control and management of thalassemia, and encourage multi-centric randomized control trials for generating evidence-based, robust solutions which can help in planning management strategies for the patients.

SUMMARY

- Thalassemia is a common monogenic disorder worldwide and in India, causing chronic health burden and expensive lifelong treatment, necessitating improved prevention and affordable therapies.
- *Prevention research*: Carrier detection and genetic counseling, including premarital and antenatal first-trimester screening, are essential to reduce affected births. Uniform epidemiological data are needed to guide health policies.
- *Technological advances*: AI-based algorithms and mobile apps are being developed to improve thalassemia screening but require validation to differentiate iron deficiency prevalent in India.
- *Challenges in prenatal diagnosis*: Current invasive prenatal diagnostic methods limit accessibility; noninvasive prenatal diagnosis (NIPD) using cell-free fetal DNA (cffDNA) and advanced techniques like ddPCR and NGS offer promise but face technical and cost barriers.
- *Management research*: Though HSCT centers have expanded, most patients rely on transfusions; optimizing antigen-matched transfusions and safe blood supply systems remains critical.
- *Iron chelation*: Research addresses challenges like iron burden assessment, drug side effects, variable pharmacokinetics, adherence, cost, and access, aiming to improve compliance and outcomes.
- *Novel therapies*: Drugs inducing fetal hemoglobin (HbF) expression—hydroxyurea, thalidomide, short-chain fatty acids, DNA methylation inhibitors, and erythroid maturation agents like Luspatercept—show benefits but need more safety and efficacy data.
- *Curative approaches*: Allo-HSCT is limited by donor availability and risks; gene-editing therapies using CRISPR/Cas9, ZFN, and TALENs are promising but require further research to enhance efficiency and delivery.

REFERENCES

1. Soteriades S, Angastiniotis M, Farmakis D, et al. The need for translational epidemiology in b thalassemia syndromes: A Thalassemia International Federation perspective. Hematol Oncol Clin North Am. 2023;37:261-72.
2. Das R, Saleh S, Nielsen I, et al. Performance analysis of machine learning algorithms and screening formulae for β–thalassemia trait screening of Indian antenatal women. International Journal of Medical Informatics. 2022;167:104866.

3. Constantinou CG, Karitzi E, Byrou S, et al. Optimized droplet digital PCR assay on cell-free DNA samples for non-invasive prenatal diagnosis: application to beta-thalassemia. Clinical Chemistry. 2022;68(8):1053-63.
4. Gallarda JL, Dragon E. Blood screening by nucleic acid amplification technology: current issues, future challenges. Molecular Diagnosis. 2000;5:11-22.
5. Reddy PS, Locke M, Badawy SM. A systematic review of adherence to iron chelation therapy among children and adolescents with thalassemia. Ann Med. 2022;54(1):326-42.
6. Far MA, Fard AD, Hajizamani S, et al. Thalidomide is more efficient than sodium butyrate in enhancing *GATA-1* and *EKLF* gene expression in erythroid progenitors derived from HSCs with β-globin gene mutation. Int J Hematol Oncol Stem Cell Res. 2016;10(1):37.
7. Jain M, Chakrabarti P, Dolai K, et al. Comparison of efficacy and safety of thalidomide vs hydroxyurea in patients with Hb E-beta thalassemia - a pilot study from a tertiary care Centre of India. Blood Cells Mol Dis. 2021;88:102544.
8. Anurathapan U, Hongeng S, Pakakasama S, et al. Hematopoietic stem cell transplantation for severe thalassemia patients from haploidentical donors using a novel conditioning regimen. Biol Blood Marrow Transplant. 2020;26(6):1106-12.
9. Cosenza LC, Gasparello J, Romanini N, et al. Efficient CRISPR-Cas9-based genome editing of β-globin gene on erythroid cells from homozygous β039-thalassemia patients. Mol Ther Methods Clin Dev. 2021;21:507-23.
10. Locatelli F, Lang P, Wall D, et al; CLIMB THAL-111 Study Group. Exagamglogene Autotemcel for transfusion dependent β-thalassemia. N Engl J Med. 2024;390:1663-76.

Index

Page numbers followed by *b* refer to box, *f* refer to figure, *fc* refer to flowchart, and *t* refer to table.

T

U

V

W

X

Y

Z